THE Celebrity FIT CLUB WEIGHTLOSS PROGRAMME

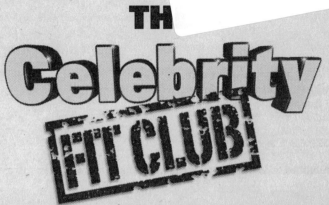

Annie Ashworth and Meg Sanders

First published in Great Britain in 2002 by
Michael O'Mara Books Limited
9 Lion Yard, Tremadoc Road
London SW4 7NQ

© Granada Media 2002.

Published in association with Granada Commercial Ventures.
'Celebrity Fit Club' is an LWT production for itv1.

Annie Ashworth and Meg Sanders are the Authors of this Work and
have asserted their right, under the Copyright Designs and Patents Act
1988, to be identified as Authors of this Work.

A CIP catalogue record for this book is available from the British Library

ISBN 1-84317-010-8

1 3 5 7 9 10 8 6 4 2

Designed and typeset by Design 23

Photographs by Ken McKay © Granada Media Group Ltd

Colour plates section designed by www.glensaville.com

Printed and bound in Britain
by Cox and Wyman, Reading, Berks

CONTENTS

Annie Ashworth and Meg Sanders are a very experienced writing/ editing partnership. Their work includes features for national magazines, development and research for Maverick TV, writing for the Web and books including the *Trade Secrets* series, *How to Beat the System* (both Orion), titles for *The Good Web Guide* and *Change Your Life with Fat Club* (Granada).
They both live in Warwickshire.

Acknowledgements
Our thanks to Sasha Jeffrey, *Celebrity Fit Club* director for allowing us to muscle in on the filming, and to Susanna Wadeson, Head of Books at Granada Commercial Ventures for having the patience of Job. Recipes reproduced by kind permission of Adam Palmer, Champneys and Orion Publishing.

INTRODUCTION

The recipe: Take eight overweight celebrities, give them the undivided attention and expertise of three weightloss professionals, film them for six months and see what happens.

ITV1's *Celebrity Fit Club* was an innovative project which proved that weight problems can be beaten for good. It wasn't about quick fixes. It wasn't about crazy fad eating plans. It was about the simple fact that eating healthily and exercising regularly will solve anyone's weight problems forever.

The celebrities who followed the straightforward advice of the experts succeeded. Those who didn't failed. It was as simple as that: they had found the elusive key to lasting weightloss and improved health. The great news is that you don't have to be a soap star, politician or a radio DJ to share the secret. It's all here for you, and the programme couldn't be easier to follow.

The magic formula

It is very likely that this isn't the first weightloss book you have picked up – your bookshelves may even be groaning with glossy, promise-all publications that you've tried to follow and relegated to an ever-growing pile of costly and depressing failures. Your dieting history may go back years. In fact 14 million of us in the UK are all trying to shift pounds at any one time, and

90 per cent of us will fail. If we haven't already thrown the books aside in hunger and frustration, the chances are that within a year we will almost certainly have put back on any weight we successfully lost. Sometimes we'll end up even heavier than we were before. How depressing is that?

But here's the good news: take on board the messages of *Fit Club* and this will be the last weightloss book you'll ever need.

Why we need to lose weight

It is just as well that 14 million of us *are* making an effort to lose weight, because we certainly need to. Weight problems have reached epidemic levels. As usual the US leads the way, but we are not far behind. In the UK, one in two of us is overweight, and one in five of us is actually obese (the term for being over-weight to a point where your health is threatened), and cases of obesity have tripled in the last twenty years.

There are an alarming number of medical conditions which are a direct result of excess weight, and they are costing the economy £2.5 billion every year. GPs like our *Fit Club* doctor, itv1's Chris Steele, have waiting rooms filling up with people who have developed:

High blood pressure
Osteoarthritis – pain and damage in the ankles, knees, hips and spine
Osteoporosis – brittle bones
Bad backs
High cholesterol levels

*Gall stones – which cause severe abdominal pain
(biliary colic)*
*Hiatus hernia – causing heartburn and indigestion.
If left untreated, can increase the risk of cancer of
the gullet*
Hernias in the groin area
Impotence
Infertility

But these are nothing compared to the killer diseases
obesity can cause. These include:

Strokes   *Heart disease*
Cancer   *Diabetes*

The **cancer** statistics are terrifying and are something
none of us should ignore:

• *40 per cent of all cancers can be prevented by eating a
low-fat diet.*

• *Cancers prevalent in obese people include breast, bowel,
prostate and ovarian.*

• *Obese women are 50 per cent more likely to die from
breast cancer than women of a healthy weight.*

Diabetes in overweight patients is perhaps the biggest
concern for the medical profession. There are two
types, I and II, and it is type II, often called maturity-
onset diabetes, which is linked with obesity, when the
body's cells don't react to insulin. Obese men and
women are twenty-seven times more likely to get type
II diabetes, and as Chris Steele says, 'It is not just a bit
of sugar in your blood, it's a very nasty disease.'
Symptoms include blindness, kidney failure, gangrene

in the lower limbs, impotence, hypertension, heart attacks and strokes. Diabetes can affect almost any organ in the body, and will undoubtedly take ten years off your life expectancy.

This is a national crisis and is causing massive concern to Paul Trayhurn, Professor of Obesity Biology at Liverpool University (the fact that a chair of Obesity Biology has been created at all shows how serious the epidemic has become). '1.4 million people are currently diagnosed as having types I and type II diabetes in this country,' he says, 'but that will double in ten or fifteen years to 3 million, due to the rise in obesity and type II diabetes.' The financial implications are dramatic. 'We spend £5 billion annually treating diabetes – so it will be double that by 2012. That really hits me in terms of the diabetes and obesity problem.'

For an entirely preventable disease, this is a crazy situation.

Why has it happened? The (big) bottom line

The irony is that the average British adult consumes 1900 calories per day, whereas fifty years ago we ate 2500. Yet half of us are now overweight. How did that happen? 'Inactivity is the culprit,' says Chris Steele. Unfortunately the advantages of our wonderfully high-tech world – cars, escalators, remote controls, computers, Playstations – all anchor our bottoms to our chairs. We've become lazy, taking only a fraction of the exercise we used to, simply because we don't need to. We can call for our food to be delivered, watch TV all evening, jump in the car to nip down to the shops.

Chris has a graphic statistic: 'Twenty-five per cent of all car journeys are less than two miles.'

Diet too plays a big part in making us bigger. Instead of the meat and two veg diet of the 1950s, we are now consuming foods that are high in saturated fat and carbohydrate, particularly the highly refined types so common in fast and snack foods: curries, burgers, crisps, chips, pasta and pizza, sweets and chocolate bars, fizzy high-sugar drinks. As a nation we eat more snacks than any other country in Europe. It's a vicious circle. The choice of these foods is enormous, so the demand for them grows. The fast, convenience food chain sector is now worth over £2.7 billion per year, and the UK market for biscuits, chocolates, and sugar confectionery is now worth £7.43 billion per year.*

How ironic that the medical profession is trying so hard to help us to live longer, and we are eating ourselves into early graves.

But what does all this mean to you?

If you are overweight, all the statistics and facts in the world will mean nothing unless you really understand and accept how your health will be affected. You *can* change the situation. You *can* achieve a healthy weight. But doing so will involve commitment on your part. Are you ready for that? If the health implications mean nothing to you at the moment, let's get a bit more personal.

Statistics from the Food and Drink Federation Food Service Report, and the Biscuit, Cake, Chocolate and Confectionery Alliance.

Be honest. Think hard about what being overweight means to you:

• Do you feel uncomfortable in your clothes?
• Do you find it hard to find clothes that fit in high street shops?
• Are you tired and lethargic all the time?
• Do you dread the summer because it means taking off clothes?
• Do you avoid looking in the mirror?
• Is it an effort to do simple things like getting in and out of the car or walking upstairs?
• Do you make jokes against yourself to get in first before other people do it?
• Do people tease you or comment on your weight gain?
• Has exercise become difficult because of your weight?
• Are you reluctant to go to a gym because of your weight?
• Do you wish you were slimmer?

If you answer yes to even one of these, then your weight is affecting your day-to-day life. Just think how much happier you could be (not to mention healthier) if you did something about it.

This is what *Celebrity Fit Club* was all about: taking busy people who had tried and failed to diet so many times before, who had fallen into bad eating habits and who had let their weight spiral out of control. They took up the challenge of making a life change and so can you!

Why those crash/fad diets didn't work

Like most of the members of *Celebrity Fit Club*, you've probably filled up on fibre, suffered (and caused others to suffer!) with the cabbage soup diet, put up with boiled eggs and grapefruit, stuck to just juice, or mixed up meal replacement powders. You may even have rolled in volcanic ash (well, Jono Coleman did!). Wasn't it hell? And surprise, surprise, none of these faddy methods actually worked. Diets by their very nature are a temporary fix. Forgive yourself for failing. There was no way you could succeed with these sort of regimes.

The reason these diets are enticing is because they promise quick results, and sometimes deliver them – but only temporarily. That's why the diet industry is worth £1 billion a year in the UK. Most work on the principle of dramatic calorie-cutting. Your body responds by using up the carbohydrate (known as glycogen) which is stored in water in the body. The scales show the pounds are going – hurrah! – but what you haven't lost is any fat. Now your body starts to panic. As far as it is concerned you are in starvation mode, and suddenly the weight loss grinds to a halt. You are left hungry, tired and fed up. You say 'what the heck', start eating 'normally' again, and the weight very rapidly goes on again (see Chapter 4 to find out more about why this happens).

Crash-exercise doesn't work either: we are inspired by pop stars and actors who have re-sculpted their bodies (conveniently forgetting that these people often have personal trainers galore). We enthusiastically join gyms in the hope that we'll get fitter just by signing the membership form and doing a session a week, and veg out for the rest of the time. Unsurprisingly, we don't see the results we were hoping for, and soon lose interest. The fact is that, of those of us who join up, one in five wastes more than £1000 a year belonging to a gym and never going. But actually cancelling your membership feels like an admission of failure. What you need is the motivation and there are plenty of tips to help you in Chapter 5.

Why *Fit Club* will work

Other diets and gym regimes have failed because they haven't provided you with a realistic plan for life – one you can sustain and live with happily. Is life really worth living if you are never allowed to eat bacon, mayonnaise, chocolate? With *Fit Club*, no food is banned and any activity is good activity. What's more you'll have energy throughout the day – no more mid-morning binges or post-lunch slumps – and a zest for life you thought you'd lost forever.

The *Fit Club* principle is so simple it will make you wonder why you've struggled all these years. Sustained weightloss is based on a three-pronged attack:

• *The motivation to become healthier and fitter*
• *Eating healthy, appetizing and satisfying food*
• *Becoming more active*
  That's it!

What the *Fit Club* was all about

The celebrities who took part in *Fit Club* met up at Champneys, the luxurious health resort in Hertfordshire, for just one day a month over a period of six months. The idea of this was to:

- *Meet with the team of experts*
- *Have their weight monitored*
- *Introduce them to exercises that they could easily fit into their lives*
- *Keep track of their exercise attainment with a stamin a assessment*
- *Give them advice on healthy eating to fit their lifestyles*
- *Help them with their motivation*

Although we can't offer you a monthly visit to Champneys, nice though that would be, the following chapters give you all the information the celebrities were given, along with lots of extra help so that you can follow the *Fit Club* plan for yourself. You'll find chapters on creating your own personal profile, finding and maintaining your motivation, exercise ideas, healthy eating suggestions for all situations, mouthwatering recipes from the Champneys' chef, answers to common questions, and lots of hints and tips along the way to help you regain control of your life.

CHAPTER 1

WHO WAS AT FIT CLUB?

A crucial element of *Celebrity Fit Club*, which put it ahead of many other health and weightloss regimes, was that members had access to the expertise of three professionals: a GP, a doctor specializing in nutrition, and a fitness instructor. Each member was given a thorough health assessment – something which is advisable for anyone wanting to lose weight or get fit – and a comprehensive lifestyle analysis. The combined experience of these experts meant that each member had a bespoke eating and exercise regime to help him or her to address and beat their weight problems.

THE EXPERTS

Harvey Walden

Any viewer who tuned into itv1's *Fat Club* earlier in 2002 will be familiar with the inscrutable Gunnery Sergeant Harvey E Walden IV. A professional soldier in the US Marines, based here in the UK, Harvey's role is to take in hand the new recruits and turn them into effective soldiers. He's the perfect man for the job: single-minded, determined, committed. His military 'failure is not an option' attitude worked extremely well at *Fat Club*. Though many of the members started out hating him, by the end they all had a grudging respect for the man who had cajoled, motivated and, at times, almost bullied them into getting up and exercising.

Born in Chicago, Illinois, thirty-six-year-old Harvey

joined up in 1985, an unusual move when there was no military history in his family. He claims he was lured into it 'because the Marine recruitment officer was the only one who had popcorn on his stand', but, in fact, his decision to become a Marine is really no surprise. The Marines epitomize the schoolboy image of soldiers: disciplined, supremely fit, uncompromising. One of the *Fat Club* members neatly summed up Harvey: 'He's Action Man made flesh'.

Harvey's tour in the UK is now over and he has moved back, with his wife Sherry and children Tiyauna (13) and Harvey V (9), to Quantico, Virginia, to welcome a new set of unsuspecting Marine recruits. His last job here was to work with the celebrities at the *Fit Club*. Being American, he had never heard of the members before meeting them on day one. To him they were not familiar personalities in politics, on TV soaps or radio programmes. They were simply people who had let their weight spiral out of control and who needed to readdress their lifestyles completely.

More familiar with working with moderately fit and committed eighteen-year-olds in the Corps, his experience with *Fat Club* was invaluable in helping him motivate middle-aged, British TV personalities: 'I learned that some people just don't realize how bad a shape they are in when they do not exercise. It really is a matter of life and death. They just take for granted the good things in life, and do not realize that exercise does not have to be hard or very difficult, nor does it have to be a chore. It's simply a way of life – just like you get up in the morning and brush your teeth or feed your face, you can partake in some form of exercise just as easily.'

He is convinced that we have slipped into bad habits because of the way we live today: 'It's very unfortunate that overweight people have got into such a comfort zone, and refuse to leave it unless you pretty much demand that they do, or give them some form of motivation to boost their self-esteem. They need some sense of accomplishment and achievement, as well as some outstanding weightloss results.'

If anything, he found the celebrity group harder to handle than the *Fat Club* members: 'Some of them really want you to hold their hand for the most part and practically do everything for them. If you could lose weight for them they would be happy. They aren't keen to leave that comfort zone, and some have the mentality that if they don't want to do something, they don't have to. They will throw a tantrum like a toddler just because they are celebrities.' In Harvey they had met their match.

Dr Chris Steele

Chris has been the resident doctor on itv1's *This Morning* programme since it began fourteen years ago. A warm and friendly north-easterner, fifty-seven-year-old Chris was born in Wallsend-on-Tyne, but has worked as a GP in South Manchester for thirty-two years. He lives close by with his wife Monica, a midwife, and four children, Anne Marie, Catherine, Matt and Andrew.

His special interest is in helping people to give up smoking – he runs one of the biggest and longest running smokers' clinics in Europe – and he has worked extensively in the media lecturing internationally on the subject. But as nearly 50 per cent of smokers put on weight when they give up, he has gained a great deal of experience in weight-management programmes. His everyday work in his surgery has also highlighted the extent of the obesity problem we now face. 'I've noticed the increase in obesity over the years, especially in teenagers and children, and seen an increase in heart attacks, strokes, cholesterol levels, diabetes and osteoarthritis. Obesity has the same mindset as smoking – it's a dependency but this time on the wrong foods in the wrong quantities.' Unlike smoking, which is a chemical addiction to nicotine, Chris acknowledges that the reasons for being overweight may run very deep psychologically, but he is certain from where the motivation to change must emanate. 'I can offer the solution, and help you and support you. The rest is up to you.'

Chris is very enthusiastic about the *Fit Club* ethic. 'The real benefit is that it will affect lots of people. They'll look at these celebrities and say, "If they can do it, so can I". It's the 'sleeper' effect. They may not act on it right away, but it's always at the back of their mind.' The excuses and explanations for being overweight given by the *Fit Club* members are no different from those he hears from patients everyday, but he says: 'Celebrity clout is powerful and the programme will be a great public health message – better than anything the Department of Health can do.'

Dr Adam Carey

Adam Carey's experience makes him an ideal choice for *Fit Club*. Not only is he a highly qualified medical doctor with a string of research projects and years of clinical experience behind him, he is also nutritional advisor to the rich and famous, so is used to dealing with celebrities and their particular foibles. His past clients include film actors, Olympic athletes and members of the Royal family. He is also currently the nutritional coach for the England Rugby team and Bolton Wanderers Football Club, helping them to tailor their diets to optimize their performance and health.

Although the physical demands asked of the *Fit Club* members were not as extreme as those asked of, for example, Angelina Jolie in her role as Lara Croft in *Tomb Raider*, they were certainly challenging in other ways. Fortunately, Adam's impeccable research background gave him an authority with the celebrities that was sorely needed at times, as he coaxed them to change their entrenched habits and doggedly held, but often misguided, beliefs on the subject of nutrition.

Adam trained as a Gynaecologist and Obstetrician, and has a special insight into the kind of problems that face women as they grapple with hormones and weight, both during and after their reproductive years. His experience as a physician and nutritionist has led to his absolute conviction that 'maintaining a healthy weight by means of balanced, intelligent nutrition and regular exercise is absolutely essential for everyone, both as a means of preventing disease and of coping with it when it occurs'.

No stranger to the media, Adam is a frequent contributor on radio, TV news and documentaries, and also writes for sports magazines and the national press. He sees *Fit Club* as a fascinating and much needed way of bringing the topics of nutrition and health into public debate. 'This was always going to be a very interesting and intense experience for the celebrities, and I admire them all for doing this on national television. Many people find it very difficult to make these changes and often at the end of the first month, they've done little or nothing apart from think about it. But this programme is being made over a six-month period so it focuses everybody's attention into that period.'

Despite his intensive programme of work and research, Adam finds the time – and energy – for regular exercise, particularly his passion for watersports, including sailing, diving and windsurfing, and being married to a doctor and the father of two young children, he is ideally qualified to show the celebrities how to juggle the demands of family life, work and leisure.

THE CELEBRITIES

Jono Coleman

The bubbly voice of Heart FM's breakfast show, Jono Coleman is the classic fat, funny man. Though born and bred in North London, he emigrated with his family to Sydney when he was eight and despite having lived back here for many years, still has that appealing Aussie twang to his voice. Affectionately known by his wife Margot as 'Johnny Neckless', on account of his double chins, he's a regular on TV and will be familiar to readers of *Punch* and the *Evening Standard* as a restaurant reviewer – the ideal job for a man who admits he simply 'loves food'.

Jono has never been what he calls 'a six-pack man'. Chubby from childhood, he became an expert at copying his mother's handwriting to forge letters excusing him from games lessons at school. 'I was always worried when we had PE classes – and there was a lot of that in Australian schools. One team kept their shirts on, the other took theirs off. I always wanted to be in the team that kept theirs on because I had sort of "man breasts" even as a little boy... I remember getting fatty taunts. I think part of the reason why I became the court jester in the classroom – the one who made the teachers and the students laugh – was because it was a way of not getting bullied in the playground.'

His teenage years were just as bad, and his mother took him to see a doctor who prescribed a thousand-calorie-a-day diet – agony for the ravenous Coleman. 'My mum had to make my lunches for me so when all the other kids, all the little Italian and Greek kids, were eating salami sandwiches and big chunks of cheese, I was sitting there with a little piece of Dutch cheese and some Ryvita with a little bit of Vegemite.'

A burgeoning interest in girls made him address his weight problem – ' "You're just like a big brother and I love you because you are so cuddly" is just about the last thing you want to hear when you are sixteen or seventeen!' he says – and he got into diet pills (Durmamine) which, he claims, did nothing but put him in a foul mood. Instead he rebelled against the

Australian Bondi Beach body-beautiful mentality: 'If you wanted to be really counter-culture and to be cool and chilled, you didn't get into sport. I knew that Jonathan Coleman wasn't destined to be an Olympic runner. Maybe an Olympic eater.'

Lack of sport in his life – in fact lack of exercise of any kind – was just one reason behind his large weight gain over recent years. 'My weaknesses are probably to do with my lifestyle,' he said before starting *Fit Club*, 'having to get up at five o'clock in the morning for the breakfast show, then eating a little bit too much breakfast because you haven't had anything earlier in the morning.' The Heart FM canteen provides what he calls 'very dangerous things – sausages, scrambled eggs, bacon, hash brown potatoes. And then there's that whole thing of "Hey, what are you doing for lunch?" I love food. I love nothing more than going to a restaurant with friends and ogling the wine list. I love red wine. I love white wine. I'm not huge on desserts, but if someone else is having one, suddenly I find myself with a piece of pecan pie in front of me. And there are sandwiches on a table at a meeting, or if I'm in a shop buying a paper and the kids say, "Can you get me an ice cream?" nine times out of ten I'll buy one for myself as well.'

Jono admitted too that, in the evening, he would polish off the remains of his children's tea, then he and his wife, Margot, might drink a couple of bottles of wine. Alcohol is a high source of calories, which is easy to forget, and would undo all the good of Margot's healthier suppers. Jono's other downfall was the car – Margot had even known him drive to the corner shop – and it didn't help that he was collected by a radio station car in the morning and dropped home afterwards.

'He doesn't actually eat a huge amount more than most men. He doesn't exercise. He avoids any sort of excess movement at all,' said Margot when asked about her husband's lifestyle. 'He doesn't like going to the top floor of our house to say goodnight to the kids. He'd rather have them kiss him goodnight downstairs. He's cumbersome now so he avoids exercise. It's a compounding thing.'

It's not that Jono hadn't made an effort in the past. He was a typical yo-yo dieter, and claims to have tried everything, from a personal trainer and Weight Watchers to some pretty drastic measures: 'I've been on lots of different fad diets over the years. I've lost weight and put it back on again. One diet involved just fasting, one just having juices, one just soup – I lost quite a lot of weight but I got very, very bored. Then there was one where I used to have an injection in the bottom and it was like a cow's urine or something like that! I had all sorts of really stinky seaweed rubbed all over, and I had one thing in Japan once where you were actually buried in volcanic ash.'

'I think it's down to you and the knife and fork.'

Jono was fully aware of why these types of diet regime didn't work. 'They're things you can't really build into your lifestyle. You need to change the way you do things. I think it's the actual lifestyle changes that is the bit that never really clicked in my head.

I've tried them all but I think it's down to you and the knife and fork.'

Even before joining the other members at the *Club*, he had the information in his head about what he needed to do and, if he was honest, knew that exercise was a critical part of the weightloss equation, but somehow the motivation hadn't been strong enough. So what was different this time?

One incentive was a Gucci jacket he bought a few years ago. 'It was a hell of a lot of money and I can't do it up anymore. My aim is to get back to the stage where I can actually fit back into it.'

But his real reasons for joining *Fit Club* ran much deeper. There is a family history of heart attacks. Jono's grandfather had heart disease and his father died in his early sixties. Jono was aware of the genetic risks, and his fear was that he would follow the same pattern. 'I've never been this heavy. It's that fear of thinking that if I don't do something now... I'm not going to be this indestructible guy that just keeps on going. I don't want to die. I've got two young children and I want to be there at their twenty-first birthdays. I look at myself on television, and I just think that I look fat and it's not a pleasing picture. The next time I want to see myself on television looking healthier and being a good example to my kids and to other kids. The reason I decided to do the show, after much apprehension and soul searching, is the fear of dying, the fear of getting sick. The fear of finding out that I am not some sort of superman.'

From the start his willpower was strong: 'There are lots of temptations, but they are not insurmountable,' he said at the beginning. 'It's just a question of using that little bit of willpower that I've stored away round the back here somewhere. I've done it before and I'll do it again.' The challenge for Jono was changing his whole lifestyle around the confines of his job, and finding a way to make that change permanent.

The Experts' view of Jono

All the experts were concerned by Jono's starting weight which fell into the Morbidly Obese category on the Body Mass Index (see pages 56-57 for an explanation of this). In the opinion of both Adam Carey and Chris Steele, this put him at an extreme risk of developing diabetes and, combined with the family history of heart disease, made a heart attack or stroke before the age of sixty highly likely.

Harvey was encouraged by his awareness of the health risks and his determination to live long enough to see his children grow up, but Adam Carey was not fooled by Jono's wisecracking personality. 'He uses his sort of jokey, light-hearted attitude to life about himself. He thinks it's fine to be this size – it's quite funny – but deep down he knows it's not really funny. You wonder if it's a protective mechanism. I think there is an awful lot of tension at home about this issue. His wife is very supportive so I think that he's got things set up in the right way now. I think he will lose two stone just doing the dietary changes, but my real concern is that he's a zero-exerciser. Adopting exercise patterns that he can carry on in the longer term is going to be the secret of his success.'

Ian McCaskill

Now retired, sixty-four-year old Ian McCaskill was, for many years, the avuncular Scottish frontman of the BBC weather forecast. His happy, bespectacled face – so hilariously mimicked by *Spitting Image* – would take the sting out of forecasts of gales and blizzards. Ian actually tried to buy his puppet at the Internet auction – it was too expensive – probably because he has been described as the 'only person to have looked worse than his puppet'!

But inside that portly figure beat the heart of a man who wanted once again to be the slim, good looking teenager who wowed the girls. 'At university (in Glasgow) I used to cox for the rowing crew,' he said. 'I was eight stone.' After two years' National Service in the Royal Air Force Meteorological Corps from 1959, he joined the civil service in the Met Office in 1961, working all over the country and ending up at the London Weather Centre. He eventually joined the BBC in 1978. He reckoned that, since those heady days of RAF uniform and dapper moustache, when he could demolish chips and haggis without putting on an ounce, his rise in weight had also been meteoric, piling on a stone every decade. 'It might not sound like much,' he said, 'but the trend had been constantly upwards.'

The culprits? Success and the BBC canteen. 'Civil servants don't make much money, but on telly you make a bit more, so I started eating on a regular basis and my weight went up.' He blames good Corporation grub as the reason why, on European weather broadcasts, his physique obscured Portugal!

Despite the health benefits, he admitted too that giving up smoking in 1997 (after two previous attempts) resulted in a big weight gain. 'Smoking kills your appetite stone dead. I gave up and put on two stone because you've got to do something. You either kick nuns or you eat more, and I was fed up with kicking nuns.'

'I go to the supermarket every day just for samples of cheese, and stuff them in. I pretend I'm not actually eating them.'

Though he tried to eat good food, with plenty of organic food in his diet, his weakness was the added extras: 'I'm afraid I do like biscuits,' he said sheepishly early on at *Fit Club*. 'I try to avoid cheese, but I don't manage it completely.' In fact deeper investigation revealed a closet cheese fanatic: 'I go to the supermarket every day just for samples of cheese, and stuff them in. I pretend I'm not actually eating them.' He was particularly fond too of pub food, and has joked in the past that he attempts to keep both pubs in his Buckinghamshire village profitable, and despite trying to choose healthy options, admitted that most meals came with chips.

Alcohol, too, was an issue. Though he knocked drinking spirits on the head about twenty years ago, he admitted to a weakness for wine – 'it's the Celtic gene'– and with a good secondary career as an after dinner speaker, was faced quite often with the temptation of big corporate ('How apt!') dinners.

Ian had an extra incentive for losing weight. Four

years ago he married Pat (his first wife died of breast cancer – and by doing *Fit Club* he is raising money for Breakthrough, the breast cancer charity). 'I think I owe it to my new wife to get back to a decent weight and look a bit better. I actually want to hang around for a bit – I don't want to die at sixty-five and go to the great chip fryer in the sky. I want to go on and do nice happy things. Basically I want to be fitter, not just lighter.'

His exercise regime was far from disgraceful, but he was probably not doing enough of the right sort. 'I've spent forty years avoiding exercise. I'm lazy but cunningly conceal the fact. I do swim once or twice a week, but swimming is not very good for your shape. I mean, have you ever seen a slim walrus? I do love walking, especially with my wife, but I've got to do a bit of structured exercise. Not jogging, though. Jogging is boring and I will not be bored. I left it to Harvey to come up with something imaginative.'

Like many of us, Ian has been down the diet route before, with a moderately successful stab at Weight Watchers some years ago, shifting about a stone and a half, but his motivation failed. 'I stopped doing it, didn't I? It wasn't enough of a lifestyle. It's really got to be a lifestyle thing.'

Though not fiercely unhappy about the way he looked, Ian had a medical reason for needing to lose weight. 'I suppose if I was lighter I could walk further and run faster, but I do have a slightly elevated blood pressure. It doesn't worry me because the pills are great, but I wouldn't mind getting off the pills.'

Ian was enthusiastic about the *Fit Club* ethos, and

before starting the *Club* gave up alcohol completely. His aims were to 'miss out puddings, cheese and bread rolls and I'm working on the abolition of roast potatoes'. He had plenty of support from his two daughters and his wife. 'She will make sure that I eat healthily and not too much, and she will no doubt check my pockets every day to make sure that there are no little samples of cheese, Jammy Dodgers or chocolate biscuits.'

The Experts' view of Ian

Adam Carey saw Ian as typical of men of his age, whose weight has 'snuck up the scales as the years have ticked by' and who have put themselves in danger of diabetes. 'The interesting thing is that we have measured the percentage of his body that is made up of body fat and it's about 37 per cent – the normal range is between 15 and 20 per cent – so he is almost twice as fat as he should be. He is not overweight' – a reasonable target of weight loss for Ian over the course of the *Fit Club* would be two stone –'so his programme needs to be very exercise-driven.' He admired Ian's motivation however – he'd shown strength before in giving up drinking and smoking – and was not concerned that Ian wouldn't absorb dietary messages he is given. 'He's one of those guys that once he's decided something, he'll be able to get out and do it.'

Harvey Walden felt Ian needed to be cautious of over-exertion in view of his age, especially as he seemed enthusiastic and motivated – in fact, so motivated Harvey was surprised he hadn't caught the health and fitness bug a long time ago. His challenge was to find Ian a solution to his dislike of gyms, and to devise an enjoyable fitness programme for him.

Nicola Duffett

Nicola's acting career has taken her from the refined atmosphere of Merchant Ivory's *Howard's End* to Albert Square and *Eastenders* as the hapless Nigel Bates's wife Debbie, to her current role as Kat Matthews in Channel 5's successful soap, *Family Affairs*.

She has found a niche for herself in recent years in playing characters 'who were once beautiful and have gone to seed', so ironically her weight – she wanted to lose two stone – worked in her favour when it came to winning roles. 'I'm quite lucky in a way not to be the normal, size 10, blonde, skinny actress, because often when I go up for jobs, there's only two or three other people that are going up for it. *Celebrity Fit Club* is probably going to make me get so thin and fit, I'll end up not being able to work!'

'I'm not so bothered about the way I look,' she said early on, realizing she would get very depressed if she were. TV screens notoriously gives the illusion of about 10 extra pounds in weight. 'On screen you have to see yourself all the way round. If it bothered me, I don't think I could possibly be a soap actress. In fact [the *Family Affairs* production team] are not too keen for me to lose too much weight for the part.' But a five-episodes-a-week soap can be tremendously stressful, and Nicola often comes home exhausted at the end of a tough day. 'I'm completely knackered most of the time.' For her, weightloss and getting fit would help with her stamina and give her more energy.

'I'm overweight because I like food,
because I like to eat too much.'

Like many women she was a classic yo-yo dieter and has a wardrobe full of clothes which range from size 10 to size 16. She admitted her weight varied season to season, and described herself as a 'sort of hibernating animal'. Brought up abroad in Ghana, Singapore and Malta, as he father pursued his Navy career, she craves sunshine and in the winter 'just hides under my duvet snugly and warm eating cheese and biscuits'. It was during these months that the weight piled on. Come spring, she would burst out of her chrysalis and eat healthy food, but in winter time food was fuel. 'I'm overweight because I like food, because I like to eat too much,' she said. Her weakness? Savoury foods, notably cheese and pasta. 'There's nothing I like more than a fairly creamy, cheesy bowl of pasta.' She was keen to dispel the impression that she made bad food choices all the time – 'I do eat masses of fresh vegetables, and I'm not an unhealthy eater' – but she hugely under-estimated the calorie damage of booze. Almost as an afterthought she added, 'I think, too, I have got to start cutting out the old vodkas and all the sort of sugary mixers that go with them.'

Like many actors, Nicola was, and still is, faced with the added temptations of the free studio canteen on set, and her day is wall-to-wall food. She described a typical scenario: 'We share our studios with *The Bill* and they always used to call this' – patting her stom-ach – 'the "Bill Bulge". You start off (sometimes at 7am) with a cooked breakfast – sausages, black pudding and bacon, fried eggs and mushrooms and toast. At lunchtime again, if it's really cold and you're filming outside, all you want is stodge. You know, roast beef, Yorkshire pudding and roast potatoes with lots of cabbage and gravy. Then lots of cheese and biscuits, then at four o'clock all these cakes and sandwiches come around. Then I go home and eat more cheese and biscuits really... it's not great!'

Though filming may be mentally draining, exercise it is not. Her excuse was 'last minute changes in scenes' which meant that she was unable to leave the studio to go for a run. The 'need to look at lines' was another reason for not getting out there when she could. 'By the time I get home – sometimes at eight at night – the last thing I feel like is going for a run.' But she wasn't fooling herself. 'It's a *Catch 22* situation because if you don't go for a run then you don't get fit.' For her, *Fit Club* was about finding self-discipline, but she admitted: 'I don't really have much.'

The Experts' view of Nicola

All the experts agreed that Nicola was typical of many people who need to lose weight, but will find every excuse in the book not to exercise or eat well. In the past she had been able to crash diet to lose weight for an acting role when she needed too, but she lacked the motivation to make those changes permanent. Adam Carey's initial investigations showed that, though Nicola did not need to lose more than a couple of stone, she had a body fat percentage of 35 per cent when it should be nearer 24 per cent for a women of her age. 'That would be helped by exercise, but she is not prepared to do any. She's going to struggle. When you crash diet you lose muscle mass not your fat mass. She may have been lighter as a result of diets, but when she started to eat normally again, she put back on the muscles.'

All agree that her amazingly chaotic lifestyle was the problem: 'It's a very party lifestyle, lots of alcohol and lots of eating late' and Chris Steele was unconvinced by her protestations that her body image was not important to her. 'Who in the media,' he said, 'would admit that their size and shape was not important?'

Kay Purcell

Kay is as feisty in real life as Cynthia Daggert, the character she plays in *Emmerdale*. Fun and friendly, Kay has a big personality, and though she has said, 'I love being big', having been large all her life, she realized that she was actually becoming too big. 'I'm not fit and I'm big and I'm going to kill myself. I'm uncomfortable with it too... I've really been struggling with my weight in terms of how I feel about myself, and I suddenly realized I couldn't get into clothes that I was wearing. It's soul destroying. I thought, God I'm actually getting out of control with it.' She found that her weight was even beginning to affect her ability to do simple things, like going upstairs or playing with her children Ashley (17) and Shemar (4).

'At teatime it's cakes, cream cakes, and I just can't say no. You can't resist them, can you?'

'I've got to get back to being more physically active.

I want to lose weight to give myself more energy.' Energy is something she needs in bagfuls. Like Nicola, Kay works to a demanding filming schedule which is mentally draining, but involves little physical activity, and has the additional temptations of that studio canteen. A typical day is a catalogue of culinary disaster: 'I'm in the studio for 7 o'clock, so I've not got time to organize anything and, well, I'm disorganized anyway. So it's a fry-up, then we have a break at 11 o'clock-ish and it's coffee and biscuits and I'm hungry. Then there's a choice at lunchtime and it's stuff that's not particularly healthy – like meat pies. In between times it's a very sedentary life. At teatime it's cakes, cream cakes, and I just can't say no. You can't resist them, can you? I know what I'm doing is bad, but it's a question of trying to stop that.'

In her home life, Kay was eating all the wrong things too. If her Jamaican husband, Cheddie Jarrett, didn't cook – and if he did, it was usually high-fat Jamaican recipes – the family would either go to the pub for a meal or call in a takeaway. 'I never cook. There are no pots and pans in the house where we live in Leeds. It's all easy, quick convenience food.' Jamaican rum and coke, too, is a particular favourite evening tipple – between the two of them, they get through a couple of bottles a week – to wash down the odd snack of crisps, chocolate and ice cream.

Part of Kay's problem may have been the confidence she claimed to have in herself and her size. 'I have never lost a part because of weight or anything like that. I don't think people would dare to tell me to lose weight because that is partly who I am... I've always been big and it's something that people have had to deal with. If they don't like it, that's tough.' Only recently had she began to understand the risks she was running with her health.

There was little pressure from home either to lose the pounds. To begin with, Cheddie found the idea of her joining the programme a joke. To give him his due, he was behind her 100 per cent once she had made the decision, but did not see weight loss as an issue. He had noticed that she was not the size 16 woman he had met seven years ago, and that finding clothes to fit was becoming harder, but qualified: 'For me her size was not a problem. I'm happy with the size she is.'

Like the other *Fit Club* members, Kay had dieted on and off in the past, including a fruit-and-water-only regime, which she described as 'hell'. The result was predictable: 'I lost the weight, but the minute I started eating again of course, I went to double the size I was.' She was more successful with Weight Watchers, but again the weight stayed off for a while until she 'started eating again'. This last statement reveals how, to Kay, diets had been about deprivation. She had chosen radical eating plans that had stopped her eating foods she enjoyed. They had been as unrealistic as the targets she had set herself.

What she needed to address, and this was where the programme could help her, was the way she was living her life as a whole. She was trapped in a cycle of routine and habit dictated by her job. In her mind she could not break the mould of being constantly surrounded by food all day and then returning home exhausted and taking the easiest option: fattening, unhealthy takeaways and an evening of little or no activity. 'Suddenly you realize,' she said, 'you have been eating all day. Maybe just stopping to breathe!'

Exercise played no part in her life at all. 'I used to so enjoy it, but it is so out of my life now that the thought of it is like hell to me.' One reason that exercise had fallen out of her routine was as a result of a slipped disc when she was pregnant with her son, Shemar. 'It put me off and made me frightened of doing anything. That was the steady decline into doing nothing until it became much easier to go "Noooh, you know My Back"! Actually it's much better to do something, but much easier to sit and chill.'

Her weightloss motivation was to achieve a particular dress size rather than to lose a number of stones – in fact she was not keen to discover her true weight at all and hadn't stood on the scales for four years before the first *Fit Club* weigh-in. Instead she had set her heart on being a size 16 again. Her motivation was also to prove her son Ashley wrong, who observed how much slimmer she was in some old photographs. 'You'll never get back to being like that,' he challenged. The gauntlet was down and she became even more determined.

The Experts' view of Kay

Kay's weight at the beginning of the *Fit Club* showed her to be, like Jono, morbidly obese and in Adam Carey's opinion this put Kay in serious danger of an obesity-related disease such a diabetes. Chris Steele was concerned that, by never stepping on the scales, she was in denial about her weight. Adam was more concerned about her lifestyle: 'She's eating three canteen-style meals a day, and in the evening is snacking on crisps or cheesy biscuits with her favourite tipple – that could be 1500 to 2000 calories a night.'

Harvey, in true no-nonsense style, had little patience with her excuse that there was never enough time to exercise. 'All she has to do is get on the exercise bike at the set and cycle for thirty minutes. She can do this at home too while she's watching the news. There are ways around it.'

Support from those close to her was also a worry. In Adam's view she had been getting messages from friends and family that she looked great the way she was. 'She needs positive reinforcement,' he said, but there was the additional complication that the character she plays in *Emmerdale* may not be scheduled to lose weight. Adam Carey was forthright: 'If she doesn't lose weight, she won't be around to play the character.'

Rik Waller

Life has changed out of all recognition for Rik Waller since his appearance on *Pop Idol* in 2001. In the space of only about twelve months, he went from singing karaoke in country pubs around his home town of Gillingham, in Kent, to instant fame as one of the qualifying *Pop Idols*. The nation watched, enthralled, and speculation was rife over his dramatic departure – it was in fact a throat infection that forced him to withdraw – but a recording contract with EMI has secured him success. All this before his twenty-first birthday.

At the beginning of *Fit Club*, Rik was working harder

than ever before. Although he loved the creative challenges of life as a recording artist, he recognized that not all the changes were for the good. 'It's a very difficult, very demanding lifestyle. You don't get any time to have a routine and I want to put a bit of routine back into my life.'

With fourteen-hour days spent in the studio, there seemed little chance of establishing a routine, and as Rik admitted, he still hadn't hit the real big-time mayhem. He was fully aware that his enormous weight was having a bad effect on his energy levels, and that losing it would help him in that respect. He also felt a sense of responsibility that came with his new position as role model, and hoped he could encourage other obese young people to face their problems, as he was determined to do. 'I'm just going to make myself feel better by myself. More stamina, more energy and I'm going to be a positive role model for the kids.'

'I have been a victim of bullying in the past ... it's made me a lot stronger.'

His high media profile as an obese young man was important to Rik. His weight has defined most of his life so far. A large toddler, Rik became tall and stocky as a schoolboy. A very shy, withdrawn child some ten years younger than his brother and sister, from an early age he spent hours alone in his room taking solace from his two abiding interests: music and computers. He was also aware of his exceptional voice, his singing at church with his grandfather attracting attention even then.

But at school, his difference marked him out for years of serious bullying, an experience that must, despite his positive attitude, have left its mark. 'Basically the whole cause of it was my weight. It really started when I was at secondary school. I almost became robotic in the way I dealt with it. I mean I never used to listen to it, it would just, like, go straight over my head and I'd always come back with something that was really cocky and made them look like an idiot.'

The bullying became steadily more physical, with serious abuse escalating to kicking, punching, spitting, being thrown downstairs or through a door, yet he never told anyone or complained of his treatment. 'I didn't like to admit defeat or that I was weak. I never admitted it to anyone because it was kind of a pride thing. It would make me look needy.' Rik's way of dealing with the stress seems to have been to immerse himself still further in music and computer games, with comfort eating as a fall-back. The habits that led to his weight gain became ingrained, but Rik refused to see the whole experience as negative.

'In the long run it's made me a lot stronger... I think it makes me realize how hard it is to get what you want when things are stacked up against you. And I just think every single day and every single name I endured or every single punch or kick I got, it's just another lump of coal on the fire and I'm full steam ahead.'

Auditioning for *Pop Idol* took tremendous courage, and at first he was turned down but, encouraged by his parents, applied again. The rest is history. 'I had to do it for myself, but I had to do it for thousands of others who would never dare go in for an audition because they know they'd get turned down. I think it was something that had to be done.'

The row between judges Pete Waterman and Simon Cowell over Rik's weight was something he was unaware of until the programme was screened, but it certainly helped to make him one of the favourite contestants. 'It's the classic David and Goliath but this time the mountainous 6' 3" bloke wasn't Goliath. It was me, the tiny little insignificant person versus the industry.' His choice to leave the programme was a difficult one for him. 'I must admit I was shaken up by it. I was like this thorn amongst the roses and it was like "Okay what am I doing here?" I was the only big person there. And I actually tried losing weight and I lost three stone basically through starvation and lots of water. It didn't make me healthy in the long run and the ultimate price I paid was losing my voice when I needed it the most.'

'It's so easy to get hooked on the chocolate drug'

Fame suits Rik, and he thrives on the limelight now; ironic when his mother insists that he completely refused to be photographed for most of his teenage years. Being noticed was nothing new for him, so it's one aspect of sudden fame that has held no fear. 'It's funny really because before I was always noticed everywhere I went but for the wrong reasons. Now I'm noticed for good reasons most of the time so it's very encouraging.'

At 6' 3" he's certainly an imposing figure. Neither of his parents is overweight, although he says his mother diets constantly, but his grandfather was exceptionally tall at 6' 8". 'I'm not quite as tall but just as solid. It is kind of a hereditary family trait.' Rik had not weighed himself for years, and had no idea what his weight was. He maintained that he didn't eat more than most other people, although he admitted to a weakness for curry and chocolate. 'They say when you eat chocolate it releases chemicals into your body, which makes you happy temporarily, so I think that's why we have so many chocoholics. It's so easy to get hooked on the chocolate drug.'

Rik put his weight down to eating the wrong things at the wrong time, more than eating to excess, and to having a slow metabolism that led to him putting on weight when others would not – an excuse that Harvey, Chris and Adam greeted with scorn. 'With the weight he has to carry round, his metabolic rate will be higher than average, not lower!' Adam explained. 'If he made the changes we suggest, he would start to lose weight immediately.'

Rik was well aware that his eating habits were at fault. 'I do tend to snack at night when I get back from the studio or when I'm in the studio. Some days I can feel really hungry and other days I just can't be bothered to eat. I think that's half my problem; the days I don't eat my metabolism never gets a chance to start. And the days I do eat, my metabolism gets overworked, so I've got to find that happy medium. Hopefully this is going to help me do that.'

The Experts' view of Rik

Rik needed urgently to take charge of his weight problem. His obesity was at a level that posed a serious threat to his health, putting him at a very high risk of diabetes, heart disease and joint problems. His lack of energy was standing in the way of his success, and there had never been a more pressing need for him to change his lifestyle. Adam Carey was very concerned, and felt that Rik was deluding himself, 'Rik is the youngest and heaviest of our celebrities and I think for any young person to make lifestyle changes is really difficult. If we all remember back to when we were twenty, we were in the pub and no one really gave a hoot about any of this sort of stuff. He's in complete denial about his weight. He's about twice the weight he should be and, though he tells me that he eats soup and cabbage and lettuce and all this sort of stuff and never touches a takeaway, things don't match up. He really is dangerously obese and although he's only twenty-one and doesn't have any signs of disease, he certainly has signs that it's impairing his life.'

Harvey felt that Rik's youth might be an advantage. 'Being as young as he is, Rik should be able to change his lifestyle and develop some positive exercise habits, and he's got to want to do that. He could make a big change in the way he looks and feels, and it wouldn't take long to see that happening. In six months he could see a big difference, and I can guarantee he's going to like the results. His lifestyle makes it difficult for him, but that isn't an excuse – he just has to try that bit harder and fit some regular exercise into his life, but I think he needs people around him encouraging him, giving him some positive peer pressure. He's got to prioritize, organize and manage his time. He's overcome a lot of obstacles to get where he is career-wise. He just needs to apply some of that determination to improve his health and lose weight. I would hate to see him wasting his life away, but he's going to be dead before he's thirty the rate he's going.'

Coleen Nolan

There has rarely been a time when Coleen Nolan has not been in the limelight. A member of the amazing Nolan family, she made her first stage appearance at the age of two. After years touring clubs around Britain, the family got their big break on *The Cliff Richard Series* for the BBC, with Coleen at the ripe old age of nine. Performances with major singing stars, including Stevie Wonder, Perry Como, Tom Jones and the late Dudley Moore, and huge record sales have marked her career. Yet following her marriage to TV star Shane Richie, Coleen turned her back on the phenomenal success she had enjoyed, and left the band to bring up her two sons, Shane and Jake.

Coleen's struggles with her weight date back some time. 'I've always been very prone to putting weight on but when I was doing the act with my sisters, obviously we would go touring a lot so that kept it down. But even when I was what I would consider slim, I still looked bigger then the rest of them because I was taller and bigger generally. Looking back now, though, at old photos I can't believe I ever thought I was fat.'

After the break-up of her marriage, in 1999 Coleen was asked to appear as a guest on *Trisha's Celebrity*

Heartbreak and so impressed viewers with her sincerity and courage that other appearances followed: first as a guest on the ITV lunchtime chat show, *Loose Women*, then as a regular guest presenter.

In mid-2000, however, The Nolans reformed for a summer season in Blackpool after Coleen's older sister Anne was diagnosed with breast cancer. It was during this tour that Coleen met and fell in love with a session musician called Ray Fensome.

Coleen's TV career, in the meantime, was going from strength to strength. *Loose Women* transferred to a studio in Manchester and, renamed *Live Talk*, gave Coleen an opportunity to feature regularly. She went on to branch out with an evening show on the Sky Wellbeing Channel called *Girls' Talk*, a chat show with a similar format.

In June 2001, Coleen gave birth to her first daughter, and Ray's first child, Ciara, and was once more enjoying motherhood when an unexpected phone call led to yet another career change. A screen test as presenter for the ever-popular *This Morning* had been an outstanding success and she was offered the chance to prove her skills as an interviewer of wit and sensitivity with guests such as Joan Collins, Lord Attenborough, Steps and many more.

'I tend to eat on the run...'

With a busy career and a young family to look after, Coleen found she had less and less time available to cook. 'When my sister had her first baby everything she gave her was fresh and she'd be up hours preparing it and freezing it, and when Ciara came along I was straight down the supermarket.'

Coleen's eating habits left a lot to be desired – and she had become very aware of this through keeping her *Fit Club* food diary. 'I have no set pattern of when I eat. You know, even when I cook for the kids I very rarely do it for myself, because especially now with Ciara, every time I want to sit down and eat she'll need something. So I tend to eat on the run or on the go all the time and therefore I end up eating lots of snacking things: chocolate and biscuits and crisps.'

Coleen, like many mothers of young children, snacked on the food her children left. 'Oh, it's terrible. I can't believe I'm admitting to that. I do sit there and hope they're going to leave a chip or two. And then when they do, as I'm carrying it out to the kitchen to get rid of it, I'll eat it. Especially mash potato, I do like a dollop of that. Ciara's not at that age yet where I like *anything* she eats but she'll get there.'

Coleen's children are very active and slim, but like all mums, she constantly kept snack foods in the house – ostensibly for them, but often temptation proved too much for her. 'I don't want to deprive them because I've decided I'm going to go on a diet. At weekends I have a house full of kids because all their mates come and stay, and all my friends say, "no wonder they like staying at your house" because I've got what they call a chocolate drawer and a crisp cupboard and they just all come round and pig out, really.'

'I'm sick of having to wear shirts hanging outside...'

Her reasons for wanting to lose weight were typical of many women her age, 'I can go round all the time and say, "Oh, I'm happy the way I am" but I'm not. I'm not happy when I look in the mirror. I'm not happy when I got out shopping and I see fantastic clothes that I would just look vile in, which limits what you can and can't wear. I'm sick of always having to wear shirts hanging outside because I'm too fat. I look horrible if they're tucked in.'

Although she was aware of the health issues associated with being overweight, Coleen was less concerned with them. 'I don't think about health problems as much as I should. I'm doing it purely for vanity reasons. I think in the business I'm in, rightly or wrongly, it is very important how people look at you. If I get slated in the papers at the moment, which is quite frequently, it's always about my weight – you know, "fat and frumpy" – and although you can say it doesn't hurt, it does.'

Coleen had dieted before, regularly attending classes to be weighed. 'At first I thought, "Oh, how embarrassing" but it's the only way I'm going to stick with it. I think it's really good to go where you have to stand in front of people and be weighed and I lost a stone and a half on that. That was really good, but what happens is in the end you get to a certain weight when you start to feel great. Then it was just flattening out, so I was staying the same every week or not losing.' Everyone will be familiar with the scenario. She started to miss weigh-ins. Just the odd week at first then, as she admitted: 'you can't be bothered going and that's where it gradually all crept back on'.

The Experts' view of Coleen

Adam Carey recognized in Coleen a tendency he sees in many mothers of young children: 'Despite the demands of her career, Coleen is a typical mum, and in my experience mums seem to put themselves last in everything when it comes to eating, when it comes to exercise, when it comes to almost everything. I think that the big risks for Coleen are going to be over the course of the next few months; the baby is going to need a lot of looking after, the rest of the family is still going to be needing her and she's got to try and find the time to look after herself.'

The experts agreed that Coleen would need support from her family to succeed, because so many of her bad eating habits centred on the demands of the family. Adam explained, 'She doesn't have a structured eating pattern for herself because her life revolves around the children's routines. The food that she is picking up tends to be their biscuits and crisps and potatoes wedges, so she's acting as a garbage disposal unit at the moment. Her attitude is good, though. She's made the connection that if she does this for herself, it'll be good for her kids too, and that will be a powerful motivator for her.'

Harvey understood the pressure she was under, but was impressed by her determination. 'I expect her to do well. She is a self-motivator, and she shows some self-discipline during fitness training. She has that "take charge" attitude and she's definitely given 100, 110 per cent so far. She just recently had a baby, so she had some problems with not getting a babysitter and being able to go out and exercise, but I think now that she's on a mission, she has what she needs to accomplish it. I think she'll do well and she's raring for it, so she's ready to go.'

Tommy Walsh

Tommy must be Britain's most famous builder. A giant of a man at 6ft 5in, he looms large on the BBC's hugely successful Ground Force Series. While Alan Titchmarsh talks design and Charlie Dimmock wields the spade, it is Tommy who puts in the back-breaking work. He is to terracing what Delia Smith is to cranberries.

Tommy still runs his own small building business in Hackney, East London, which specializes in hard land-scaping, but fame came his way when he met the executive producer of Ground Force while doing some building work on her house. She was so impressed by his knowledge that she invited him to screen-test, and he joined the Ground Force team six years ago.

Ironically, with his TV success came a change of lifestyle and an increase in his weight. When they first met, he was, according to his wife, Marie, 'a Greek god. All strength. Perfect, really,' and hard work kept him that way. Though he was still having to put in a certain amount of physical work once he started filming, the very nature of making a programme – technical issues, re-takes, waiting around while other scenes are filmed – meant he spent far less time actually working manually.

'I work harder now than I've worked ever,' he explained on starting Fit Club, 'but it's different. You do a lot of travelling and the hours are very long. But it's not as much physical exertion as I used to put in when I was a contractor and I think there lies the problem. Although I still keep my hand in the building work outside of TV, it's just not the same. I used to be able to burn up calories quite easily years ago. If you've got a big concrete floor to spread or you're going to plaster a room out, you really get into it and you build a sweat up and then you burn it all off, but I don't do that now.'

For a man with his enormous frame, Tommy said he ate remarkably little. Unlike many builders who survive on chocolate and crisps, he seemed able to resist and claimed to consume a fairly healthy meat and two veg diet, with the odd indulgence of fish and chips, but blamed a 'slow metabolism' and age for his increasing size – both excuses which Adam Carey and Chris Steele scorn. 'I think my metabolism has slowed down so much it's actually in reverse action,' he said. 'I eat the least of everyone on Ground Force. Alan hasn't got a pick on him because he's always on the move and he burns off the extra calories that way. But with me it just 'sits up' and this is probably the heaviest I've ever been.'

He was not enjoying the change in his body: 'I feel heavy. Although my jeans are a 38 inch waist, they'd probably be a little bit better in a size 40, but I don't want to go there. If I could lose this weight, I'd like to try and keep it off.'

'I'm a builder and part of your apprenticeship is the ability to drink.'

But indulging in butter on his potatoes and the fat on his meat ('it gives it flavour'), was not the crux of Tommy's problem. His Achilles' heel was undoubtedly his penchant for booze.

'Yeah, I drink. I'm a builder and part of your

apprenticeship is the ability to drink ale. I passed my apprenticeship years ago with flying colours and I've been trying to improve my handicap every since.'

His particular weakness, however, was for Bailey's Irish Cream, which provides a staggering 320 calories per 100 ml compared to 65 for dry white wine. 'The trouble when you drink too much beer, it's a little bit sour. I crave something sweet so I started drinking Bailey's, but it's not just an ordinary shot of Bailey's. I've got this lovely crystal glass – it's just under a half pint – and I fill it up with crushed ice. The Bailey's is kept in the fridge, I pour that in and then leave it to stand for about five minutes and then drink it. The only problem is stopping at one glass.' Tommy was not doing the calculations: a pint of Bailey's was providing him with over 1700 calories.

The occasional game of football was simply not enough to counteract this level of calorie-intake, and spending much of 2001 writing his book, *Tommy Walsh's DIY Survival*, simply compounded the problem.

It was his wife who enrolled Tommy in Fit Club. At first he admitted he had reservations: 'I knew I was getting fat, but I didn't think I'd have to sort of lose weight publicly. But it's for a good cause, raising money for a kids' charity. It's a challenge for me.'

Tommy's self-imposed target was to drop a couple of stone, but he needed to get the facts straight about his eating and drinking habits, and overcome his resistance to forms of exercise Harvey would find most suitable for him. 'I'm not a great lover of training for training's sake,' Tommy admitted before meeting Harvey. 'If there's a participation sport then that's what I like to do, but running for the sake of running holds no appeal to me at all. I don't want to get bored with [the suggested training programme]. It would have to be interesting or else I probably won't be able to commit to it.'

At 46, his days as a Greek god may be over, but Tommy did acknowledge that weightloss would have its advantages. 'It will probably help me in my athletic prowess as a goalkeeper. At the moment, when it's raining and I dive across the goal, it's more like a belly flop.'

The Experts' View of Tommy

Tommy's height was deceptive, and Adam Carey's calculations were surprising. 'Tommy's not just overweight, he's actually obese (with a reading of 34 on the Body Mass Index – see pages 56-57), and he's in the top end of that range. He's carrying it well because he's a big, strong guy, but a realistic weightloss for him would be four stone during Fit Club, and he'd still have a little bit more to lose after that.'

Exercise was not the issue. As a fitness specialist, Harvey was impressed by how naturally fit Tommy was, and how 'on the assessment he took off like he was running for the Olympic trials', but all three experts were under no illusions that other areas of Tommy's lifestyle had to be addressed very seriously.

Adam Carey was blunt: 'I think the question mark, as for several of the other participants, is over alcohol. It's very difficult to compensate with exercise for taking in 2000 calories at the end of the day in the form of alcohol, because you just can't exercise that much.' Both medical doctors were concerned that Tommy is already showing early signs of cardiovascular disease. In addition to revealing medical tests, Chris Steele had noted a further heart-disease indicator: 'Research has shown that if you have a crease going across the lower ear lobe there's an increased risk, and Tommy has that crease.'

Their outlook, however, was positive. 'If he's able to moderate his alcohol intake, combine it with exercise and take on some dietary advice, he'll do famously because he's a fit strong guy.'

Ann Widdecombe

Ann is one of the best known names in politics, and she is frequently to be seen on the evening news as she holds forth with her outspoken views. At a time when politicians distinguish themselves by avoiding saying anything at all, her integrity and salty opinions make her a refreshing change and inspire admiration, albeit sometimes grudging, in the general public regardless of political persuasion.

But Ann knows what it is to be slim. 'I was 6 stone 12 until I was thirty and I have photographs which are quite unbelievable now. I could eat absolutely anything. I could eat chocolate éclairs, I could eat a huge meal. It didn't seem to matter what I ate. As I approached thirty, I suddenly put on quite a bit of weight, though I lost it again very easily. Then throughout my thirties I put on, very steadily, so that by the time I came into Parliament in 1987, I was a good 8 1/2 to 9 stone. And then throughout my forties, I again piled on a couple of stone.'

Now, at fifty-four, Ann had decided to take her weight in hand. 'I was suddenly getting backaches – not serious or prolonged ones – but it was something new.

It would be quite nice to be an absolutely glove-like standard size 12. When I was last size 12, I was 8 stone.' Her cholesterol level is also higher than it should be.

Ann's weightloss methods in the past had been radical, and this caused some worries for Adam. As her secretary, Gloria Nicholl, explained, 'Ann's from the crash-diet school. And you know when you crash-diet, it's boring, and you slow down your metabolism after the initial weight loss. You reach a plateau and you get discouraged and it just never works. Not to mention making you cranky.'

Ann's eating habits were also at odds with Adam Carey's suggestions, and this was likely to lead to some interesting conflicts. Fond of carbohydrates, she freely admitted that potatoes are her favourite food, and she positively loathed salads!

'Too much weight equals too much food'

Ann was one of the few *Fit Club* celebrities who didn't try to blame her weight gain on having a slow metabolism, yet ironically, because of her eating habits, she was probably the only one who did. 'I think a lot of people get heavier with age, even if they don't have a massive change of lifestyle. And I'm sure there are all sorts of physical explanations for that. Lifestyle is certainly part of it, but on the other hand there are plenty of people with a Parliamentary lifestyle who are not overweight, so it's no good looking for excuses.' She is characteristically blunt: 'If you're overweight, you're eating too much. Somewhere along the line I haven't kept control of what I've eaten. There's no point in making excuses and finding great physical explanations for it. Too much weight equals too much food.'

What Ann lacks is routine: 'There's no such thing as a typical day which is one of the problems and one of the reasons why I can never follow a set diet. Some days I might be very busy at the desk, and I might have nothing more than a sandwich at lunch time and soup and a sandwich in the evening. But other days I'll have two three-course meals because I've got an official lunch and an official dinner. So any endeavour with me for weightloss has got to be built on the assumption that there is no typical intake.'

'You won't find me regularly appearing at a gym. I mean, what a waste of time!'

A further obstacle to weightloss success was Ann's declared lack of interest in exercise for its own sake, and she showed no inclination to fit it into her already packed schedule. 'Everybody I know who goes to the gym either ends up injured or looks exhausted. I think it is a complete modern nonsense and I've no time at all for it. But exercise as something that is done as a by-product of pleasure, like swimming or walking – I love to walk all day on the Moors – then that is different, that is something that is worth doing. I'm not going to treat a gym as if it's a house of ill repute. I'm quite happy to go into one. But you won't find me regularly appearing at a gym. I mean, what a waste of time! I've got other things to do.'

The Experts' view of Ann

Ann's determination and single-mindedness were a mixed blessing for the experts. Adam Carey felt that her extreme methods of trying to lose weight were working against her. 'I think she could realistically lose a stone and a half during the course of the series, but at the moment her diet is very wrong. I actually think she should be eating more if she wants to continue her weightloss. Her body fat is surprisingly high, because these spells of fasting have resulted in her losing her muscle mass, and that will eventually stop her losing weight altogether. She will have to eat regularly to keep her metabolic rate level.'

The experts all agreed that Ann was unlikely to follow their suggestions fully. As Adam put it, 'If Ann starts to follow my advice, because she's hugely competitive when she's in control, she should do very well. But if she doesn't, it will be like pushing water up a hill.' Harvey agreed. 'She is such an individual, she refuses to be told anything. If I ask her to do five press-ups, she says, "Well, what do I need to do that for?" If you can't prove to her or show her that this is the way forward then she's not going to do it.'

For Chris Steele, Ann was representative of many people. 'I really can't see her doing regular routine exercise everyday. I think dieting is probably easier for her than exercising, and that will greatly reduce the effectiveness of what we are doing here.'

The *Fit Club* celebrities all had different issues. Do any of their problems match yours? To find your personal profile, turn to the next chapter.

CHAPTER 2

ABOUT YOU

Celebrity Fit Club may have revolved around people with a high media profile, but they were still mere mortals with weight problems that are all too typical. And their reasons for wanting or needing to lose weight may match yours. Are you a mum like Coleen, who can't resist picking at your children's food? Has your weight crept up on you as it has for Kay or Nicola? Like Jono, do you find you can't resist Chinese takeaways? You may even have discovered a weight-related medical condition, like Ann's high cholesterol level, or like her, have crash-dieted for too long. All the advice given by the series' experts at *Fit Club* can apply to you and your life too.

The fact that you have opened this book probably means that you know that you need to lose some weight – whether it's a little to hit your ideal weight target, or a lot because you know you are putting your health at risk. Successful and sustainable weight loss is achieved through sensible and healthy eating, exercise and, above all, the right attitude. If you really *want* to lose the weight you are already halfway to doing it.

So this chapter is all about *you*. Read through these charts, checklists and calculations to help you build up a realistic (and honest!) picture of the type of person you are. In this way you will create your own personal profile, so that you can set yourself an achievable weightloss and fitness target.

BODY MASS INDEX READY RECKONER

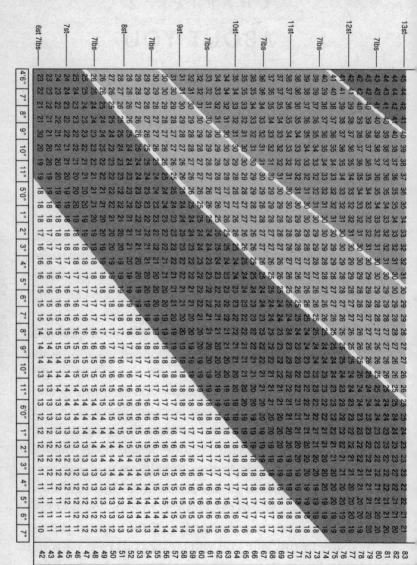

HEIGHT (Feet and Inches)

WEIGHT (Kilograms)

Very Obese
Health is seriously at risk. Losing weight **immediately** is essential

Obese
Health is at risk. Losing weight **now** should be seriously considered

WEIGHT (Stones and Pounds)

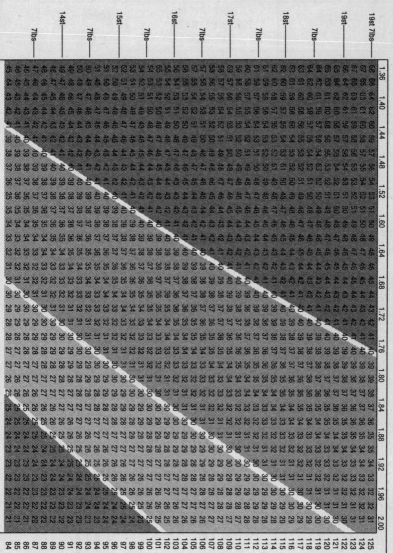

HEIGHT (Metres)

Overweight
Health could suffer.
Some weightloss should
now be considered

Healthy
A desirable BMI
figure indicating a healthy
weight

Underweight

HEIGHT AND WEIGHT CHART IN IMPERIAL MEASURES

Height	Upper limit of optimum weight BMI = 25	Obese BMI = 30
Men	weight without clothes – add 6 lbs with clothes	
5 ft 2 in	10 st 1 lb	12 st 1 lb
5 ft 3 in	10 st 4 lb	12 st 5 lb
5 ft 4 in	10 st 8 lb	12 st 10 lb
5 ft 5 in	10 st 12 lb	13 st 0 lb
5 ft 6 in	11 st 2 lb	13 st 5 lb
5 ft 7 in	11 st 7 lb	13 st 11 lb
5 ft 8 in	11 st 12 lb	14 st 3 lb
5 ft 9 in	12 st 2 lb	14 st 8 lb
5 ft 10 in	12 st 6 lb	14 st 13 lb
5 ft 11 in	12 st 11 lb	15 st 5 lb
6 ft 0 in	13 st 2 lb	15 st 11 lb
6 ft 1 in	13 st 7 lb	16 st 3 lb
6 ft 2 in	13 st 12 lb	16 st 9 lb
6 ft 3 in	14 st 3 lb	17 st 1 lb
6 ft 4 in	14 st 8 lb	17 st 7 lb
Women	weight without clothes – add 4 lbs with clothes	
4 ft 10 in	8 st 7 lb	10 st 3 lb
4 ft 11 in	8 st 10 lb	10 st 6 lb
5 ft 0 in	8 st 13 lb	10 st 10 lb
5 ft 1 in	9 st 2 lb	11 st 0 lb
5 ft 2 in	9 st 5 lb	11 st 3 lb
5 ft 3 in	9 st 8 ib	11 st 7 lb
5 ft 4 in	9 st 12 lb	11 st 12 lb
5 ft 5 in	10 st 2 lb	12 st 2 lb
5 ft 6 in	10 st 6 lb	12 st 7 lb
5 ft 7 in	10 st 10 lb	12 st 12 lb
5 ft 8 in	11 st 0 lb	13 st 3 lb
5 ft 9 in	11 st 4 lb	13 st 8 lb
5 ft 10 in	11 st 9 lb	14 st 0 lb
5 ft 11 in	12 st 0 lb	14 st 6 lb
6 ft 0 in	12 st 5 lb	14 st 12 lb

But before you start...

Although the cause of weight gain is most commonly overeating and lack of exercise, it can be caused by certain medical conditions. Dr Chris Steele suggested the *Fit Club* members asked themselves the following questions and you should too:

• Do you have any thyroid disorder or has any member of your family had a thyroid disorder?
• Are there any hormone disorders in your family?
• Are your parents or any of your sisters or brothers overweight?
• Do you take any of the following medications, which can cause weight problems?: antidepressants, tranquillizers, betablockers (used to treat heart disorders/ high blood pressure), lithium (used to treat manic depression), chlorpromazine, certain epilepsy medications, the contraceptive pill, HRT, steroids or the migraine treatment Sanomigran.
• Could you be suffering from polycystic ovary diease? This is a condition which can affect one in every five women (it is explained further on pages 69-70). As well as weight gain, this disorder can cause any one of the following symptoms: increase in facial or body hair (on the upper lip, chin, sideburn area, upper arms, upper thighs, nipple area and between the naval and pubic region), irregular periods, absence of periods, difficulty in getting pregnant, greasy skin and acne persisting beyond the teenage years.

If you suffer from any of these conditions, take any of the medications or have any of the symptoms described above, consult your GP before embarking on a weight-loss programme.

Working out your Body Mass Index (BMI) and what it should be – chart on pages 56-57

This calculation is based on your weight in relation to your height and is the best indication of how over-weight you are, unless you happen to be a fit, muscular athlete, because muscle weighs more than fat. However, the fact that you're reading this book probably rules out this scenario!

Divide your weight in kilograms by your height in metres squared (1 lb = 0.45 kg, 1 ft = 30.38 cm) [Weight kg ÷ height in m²]

For example:
A woman weighing 60 kg (133 lb) who is 1.6 m
(5ft 3 in) tall: 60 ÷ (1.6x1.6) = BMI of 23.4
A man weighing 113.4 kg (252 lbs) who is 1.86 m
(6 ft) tall: 113.4 ÷ (1.86x1.86) = BMI of 32

Rate your BMI:
Below 20   Underweight
20-25   Acceptable
25-30   Overweight
30-40   Obese
Over 40   Dangerously or morbidly obese

Your Result:...

Apple or Pear? What shape are you?

Where you store excess fat is an important factor, though no one knows why some people store it in some places and not in others. It's just the luck of the genetic draw. But doctors increasingly believe that your waist measurement is a very important indicator of your health and potential health risks.

People who carry fat around their middle (apple-shaped) rather than around their hips (pear-shaped) are more at risk of a number of medical conditions including hardening of the arteries, diabetes, high blood pressure and strokes. This is because, when fat accumulates in the stomach and waist area, it doesn't just build up under the skin. It builds up inside the entire upper torso and accumulates around the heart, liver, kidneys and intestine. It can even begin to grow inside these organs, restricting the blood flow and interfering with the way they work.

This condition is called *Central Obesity*, and the measurements are simple:

• If you have a waist measurement of over 32 inches for a woman and 37 inches for a man, you are at high risk of the diseases mentioned above.

• If you have a waist measurement of over 35 inches for a woman and 40 inches for a man, you are at a substantially increased risk.

To work out your shape, measure your waist around your belly button and hips (just below the top of your pelvis) in centimetres using a non-stretchable dress-maker's tape measure. (Take the measurement three times to get an average). Then divide your waist measurement by your hip measurement to find the ratio:

Waist in cm ÷ hips in cm = waist to hip ratio

Apple-shaped is: Female ratio of more than 0.85
Male ratio of more than 0.95

Your Result:.......................................

Your waist measurement will decrease with aerobic and toning exercise, even if the scales show that you are not losing pounds, and reducing your waist measurement by 5-10 cm can lessen the risk of developing the medical conditions mentioned above.

Dr Chris Steele has devised a simple device called the *Waist Watcher*, which he gave to all the members during the course of the *Fit Club*. It fastens around your waist like a lightweight belt and, like a tape measure, is marked out in inches and centimetres. Research has shown that dieters who used a similar device in the past lost many more inches from their waist than those who didn't, which is motivation indeed! The *Waist Watcher* shows you what happens to your body naturally (for example, a woman's waist measurement will increase with water retention just before her period) and how your waistband increases when you overeat.

As you lose weight and inches, you simply tighten the *Waist Watcher* and see that measurement diminish. The *Waist Watcher*, exclusive to *Fit Club*, is available in the shops in early 2003.

How fit are you?

Find a fairly flat piece of ground (it could be a road, park, or running track), and walk, run, or walk and run for a mile as quickly as you can without becoming uncomfortably breathless.

If it takes you:

20 minutes or over	extremely unfit
15-20 minutes	unfit
12-15 minutes	fairly fit
10-12 minutes	fit
10 minutes or under	you don't need this book!

Your Result:......................................

Ideal weights for your height: Look at the chart on page 58

Your Result:.............................kg overweight

What sort of exerciser are you?

We all have different interests when it comes to exercise. Select one of the following statements that best matches your attitudes:

• I like swimming
• I don't mind exercise but I hate getting sweaty
• I walk a short distance a couple of times a week
• I'm at home with kids so don't get a chance to exercise
• I need to exercise with other people
• I hate doing any exercise in front of other people
• I hate the gym
• I have good intentions but somehow I never get around to exercising

- My job means I am stuck in the car/office and don't get much chance to exercise
- I hate exercise and never do it

Your lifestyle

The way you live your life may be your own choice, but for most of us it's a result of juggling demanding jobs and even more demanding families. Pick the type that most describes you:

- I have just had a baby
- I am at home all day with small children
- I have a very regular routine
- I have a desk-bound job
- My job involves heavy lifting but I'm still overweight
- I spend a lot of time in the car
- I'm on my feet all day so I'm too tired to exercise when I get home
- I have a very stressful job
- I sit at a computer most of the day
- I eat out regularly on business

You and food

Our relationship with food is very complicated. Food is used to celebrate, to welcome friends, to comfort us when life is grim. Discovering how you feel about food and mealtimes will help you to understand how to control what you eat, not let what you eat control you. Pick the statements that best describe your eating habits:

- I eat when I'm hungry, grabbing food on the run
- I eat when I'm bored
- I pick from the fridge and find snacking hard to resist
- I love chocolate and treat myself to it often

- I skip breakfast but tend to eat a big meal in the evening
- I eat a lot of takeaways
- I'm busy and tend to buy ready meals
- I feed children and pick from their plates when I am hungry
- I eat when I am sad or depressed
- I have to eat out often to entertain clients and business customers
- I 'm starving when I come home from work and snack before supper time
- I like to finish a meal with a sweet taste in my mouth
- I have no willpower and will finish a packet of biscuits if it's open
- I shop for food when I'm hungry
- Eating makes me feel guilty
- I think about food all the time

Why do you want to lose weight?

You need to be honest with yourself here. A target or motivation is the secret of weightloss success.

- I feel lethargic and uncomfortable
- I've just had a baby and want to shift the extra pounds I've gained
- None of my clothes fit
- My blood pressure is too high
- There is a history of diabetes in my family
- There is a history of cancer in my family
- There is a history of heart disease in my family
- I feel embarrassed about how I look
- My back and joints ache
- I hate my appearance and can't bear to look in a mirror

Health Issues

As we said before, being overweight can be dangerous to your health in the long term. It may cause day-to-day symptoms or store up trouble for later life. Here's a list of symptoms/conditions that might indicate that you should lose weight:

Cholesterol:

Cholesterol is a sterol (a chemical precursor of natural steroids) and is not all bad news. It's made in the body, mainly in the liver, and has an important role as a building block for steroids (the sex hormones produced in the gonads and the hormones of the adrenal cortex). It's also the basis of the body's manufacture of bile salts, and is used to form cell membranes and other essential tissues. There are two forms of cholesterol-carrying proteins in the blood: high-density and low-density lipoproteins. The low-density form may promote arterial disease, and the high-density form may oppose it.

The amount of cholesterol present in the blood ranges from 3.6 to 7.8 millimoles/litre. A level above 6 millimoles/litre is considered high, and is one risk factor in arterial disease (atherosclerosis – also called arteriosclerosis), heart attacks and strokes. This is caused by plaques containing cholesterol being deposited on the walls of the arteries, reducing their inside diameter and the flow of blood. Blood clotting (as happens in the coronary arteries during a heart attack) is most likely to happen where arterial walls are roughened by such plaques.

The recommended average daily cholesterol intake

is up to 300 milligrams. People who naturally have very high levels of cholesterol (especially the low-density lipoproteins) can reduce their risk of heart attack by lowering it, by following a diet low in saturated (animal) fats, and by using cholesterol-lowering drugs.

High cholesterol foods include:

Fatty meats
Dairy products
Some poultry
Some fish
Seafood

Fruits, vegetables, grains, nuts and seeds do not contain cholesterol. The science is logical: the amount of cholesterol in the blood increases with a diet high in saturated fats. Cholesterol decreases with a diet which contains moderate amounts of unsaturated fats or oils (particularly the polyunsaturated type). These include olive oil and oily fish.

There are no specific symptoms of raised blood cholesterol, until the signs of arterial disease begin to appear, but blood cholesterol levels can be diagnosed from a simple new blood test: the cholesterol ratio. Ask your doctor for the test, especially if:

You have a family history of cholesterol disorders
There is a history of heart attacks in your family,
  especially at a young age
You are obese
You have diabetes
You have thick yellow patches (xanthomas) around
  the eyes or elsewhere on the skin
You have high blood pressure

Varicose veins:

Varicose veins are swollen, irregularly shaped veins. They are commonest in the legs, but can happen elsewhere, such as the lower end of the gullet (oesophageal varices) and in the veins from the testicles (varicocoele).

Varicose veins tend to run in families, and it is probable that there is a genetic tendency to leaky valves. But being overweight increases the risk of varicose veins, as does pregnancy, prolonged standing and local constriction from tight clothing.

Diabetes:

There are two types of diabetes, in both of which there is a loss of control over the amount of glucose in the blood. Type II diabetes, often called maturity-onset diabetes, is usually linked with obesity and is a condition in which the body's cells don't react to insulin. Type II diabetes is so closely linked to obesity that simply losing weight can reverse it.

Diabetes is diagnosed by finding sugar in the urine, and by testing the levels of blood sugar at different times of the day. As Chris Steele points out: 'People think diabetes is just about having sugar in your blood, but it's a very serious disease that can affect every organ in the body.' Diabetes that is not under control can eventually cause damage to the blood vessels. This damage especially affects the eyes, the kidneys, the circulation to the legs and the nervous system. Diabetes causes impotence in about 40 per cent of diabetic men, but thankfully this can be treated effectively with modern drugs. Diabetic disease of large blood vessels may lead to narrowing and severe interference with the blood flow. Older people with diabetes are more likely to develop bedsores and serious infections of their feet or legs, partly as a result of poor blood supply, but also because of the lack of sensation from nerve damage.

People who are overweight and over 40 are at a high risk of the disease, but Type II diabetes can be controlled by a combination of weight reduction, drugs and, if severe, insulin injections.

Back and joint pain:

This sort of pain can be a symptom of osteoarthritis, the wear and tear on the cartilage in the joints, and can be caused or exacerbated by an increase in weight on the muscles in the back, hip and knee joints. Simply by reducing the weight load, you can lessen the stress on these areas.

Polycystic ovary disease:

Polycystic ovary disease, also known as the Stein-Leventhal syndrome, is a condition associated with multiple cysts in the ovaries. The classic polycystic ovary disease features menstrual disturbances or the absence of menstruation, failure to conceive, along with obesity and excessive hair growth (hirsutism), often in a male distribution.

The exact cause is unknown, though the condition tends to run in families. Insulin resistance appears to be an important factor, especially in women who are overweight. Symptoms are greatly relieved by weightloss.

Breathlessness:

Shortness of breath is caused by excess stress on the heart (or cardio vascular system) which is having to work harder and faster to cope with extra weight, and on the lungs which have to supply oxygen to the blood. The stress on the heart will be relieved by losing weight.

High blood pressure (hypertension):

When the heart contracts, the highest pressure it produces is called the systolic pressure; when it relaxes, the lowest pressure is called the diastolic pressure. Both of these pressures are important in determining the risk of heart attack and stroke, so both will be measured by your doctor. A normal blood pressure in an adult, for instance, might be around 130/80 (often described as 130 over 80) – this is shorthand for systolic pressure of 130 and a diastolic pressure of 80. If the blood pressure is persistently high, damage to the blood vessels, including hardening of the arteries (atherosclerosis), can occur. Ultimately, this can lead to a heart attack (myocardial infarction: MI) or a stroke (cerebrovascular accident: CVA). High blood pressure causes no symptoms, so it is undetected unless the blood pressure is measured. Being overweight can increase blood pressure, but weightloss and regular exercise can reduce blood pressure.

What now?

Now you should have some idea of your BMI, your body shape, how much you should weigh for your height, how active or sedentary your lifestyle is, your relationship with food and the implications of any weight related health problems you may have.

More importantly, you have acknowledged why you have put on weight, and determined what your motivation is for losing it.

You're ready to go.

Realistic targets for weightloss – or don't be too hard on yourself!

Once you have a picture of yourself and an idea of what you need to lose, you can start your life change! But be realistic. If your expectations are too high, you will easily become de-motivated. Initial weightloss can be swift (and very encouraging!) as you lose water trapped in fat cells. But don't try to lose more than about 1 kg (2 lb) a week. Even less than that is respectable so long as the general trend is downwards. Progress will be slow but sure, and any more rapid loss will not be sustainable.

Remember that diets that make headline-grabbing promises of rapid weightloss simply do not work. They are usually very low-calorie and though early weightloss may be quick, your basic metabolic rate (BMR) – the rate at which you burn up calories – will slow down. If you lose weight rapidly through restricting your calories, especially without exercise to back it up, your BMR will drop because, in addition to fat, you will also lose some muscle.

All this makes it more and more difficult to lose weight, and then when you start eating again – as you inevitably will because you will be hungry – you will put on the weight rapidly because your normal calorie intake will exceed your body's reduced need. (See

Adam Carey's advice in Chapter 4)

Follow the advice in Chapters 4 and 5, and you'll be on the road to success.

Your Profile
Your BMI:
Your shape:
Your recommended weight for your height:
Your fitness level:
Your reasons for wanting to lose weight:

Your Targets:
BMI:
Weight:
Clothes size:
Fitness target:

CHAPTER 3

YOU CAN DO IT!

A great many diet and fitness books offer sound advice on the types of foods you should be eating and exercises you should be doing. This is all well and good, but useless if you have not found the motivation inside yourself to change your life and to stick with it.

The hardest part of losing weight and getting fit is acknowledging that you need to do something about your body. But once you have made up your mind, half the battle is over and you will achieve things you never thought possible. It's what psychologists call 'internalizing a message': you can hear and read any number of statistics about how being overweight is bad for your health, but unless it really means something to you, you will not find the motivation to do something about it.

If you have ever tried to give up smoking, you will know exactly what this means. There isn't a smoker on the planet who isn't fully aware of the dangers of smoking – there are warnings written all over cigarette packets – but until they say to themselves, 'I should give up and I'm going to do it now', they will not quit. In fact, smoking and being overweight are closely linked: when you stop smoking and lose weight, the advantages to your health are almost immediate.

The mental process is all about change. We are all bad at making changes because change can be frightening, not just because we may be comfortable with the life we live now – as Chris Steele says 'routines become entrenched' – but because change is a step into the unknown. But changes do need to be made and those changes need to be made forever. 'All I ask is that you incorporate at the very least thirty minutes' walking each day, come rain or shine,' Chris says. 'Can you invest thirty minutes a day into your future?'

So the changes are not enormous and the great thing about adjusting your life towards weightloss and fitness is that it's such a positive move. It's not unlike having a shiny new car, a whole new wardrobe of clothes, a bigger, better house. All these things make you feel better. So, too, will getting into a smaller clothes size, having more energy, feeling fitter.

Test your motivation

Chris Steele has devised an easy calculation which will show you how strong your motivation is to lose weight and get fitter. Mark your answer to the following two questions out of 10:

How **I**nterested are you in losing weight?
How **C**onfident do you feel that you can?
I + **C** = Motivation

A score of nearly 20 shows you have really come to terms with the need and the motivation to change your life. If you are interested (10 points) but unconfident (say 3 points), then you need to concentrate on your resolve, because without motivation you will not even get started.

You *can* teach an old dog new tricks!

The power of your brain is the single most important weapon in your battle to achieve a slimmer, fitter body. As children grow, their brains develop new, denser neural pathways as they learn different skills. But this pattern actually continues all our lives. Scans of adult brains show that we can alter our minds in exactly the same way as we change our bodies. By repeatedly thinking certain motivational thoughts and practising exercising attitudes – mental exercises like physical ones – we can change the way the brain works. These positive neural pathways will get stronger, and others (the ones that say, 'I can't be bothered') will get weaker.

Imagine you have to learn a new skill: it might be table tennis, computing, flying an aeroplane. With tuition and practice you will learn these new skills. The same applies to the motivation to eat differently or to exercise. Teach yourself a new mental attitude – 'I am going to eat more fruit', 'I am going to walk for at least thirty minutes each day', 'I will lose weight' – and practise it often enough, and eventually you will master it. It might be unfamiliar to start with, but very soon it will become second nature, in just the same way that you don't have to think about driving a car when you have been doing it for years. Eating an apple, taking a walk, losing weight will become part of your everyday life, like cleaning your teeth. It will no longer be difficult or a conscious effort.

Mental exercises do work, and this has been proven scientifically. Once you have the right attitude, the rest will fall into place. Here are some ideas to get you on to the right road.

Making it easier. Be honest with yourself.
Remember that *you* are the one to benefit from your
weightloss. Admit to yourself you need to lose the
weight and don't convince yourself otherwise.

**Keep reminding yourself why you have made the
decision to change your life.** If you feel your resolve
flagging, then look at pictures of yourself and again run
through the conversation you had with yourself that led
you to make the decision in the first place. Look again at
the reasons you chose in Chapter 2. You want to be fitter
and have more energy. You want to be slimmer to be able
to fit into your clothes. You want to return to the size you
once were. You want to avoid weight-related diseases
that run in your family. You want to like yourself again.

Work with someone else. If you are changing the
way you eat or starting an exercise regime, it's often
easier to have a partner or friend doing it with you.
You can bolster one another when one of you is feeling
weak or demotivated – the *Celebrity Fit Club* members
found the 'team' support invaluable. But as with an
exercise partner (see page 119), make sure your team-
mate is positive and supportive. Avoid anyone who
you think may weaken your resolve.

Set yourself a target. This might be to get back into a
particular pair of jeans, a holiday abroad or another treat
that you will allow yourself only when you reach a
certain weight. Write this and any other targets down so
that you can keep reminding yourself what you are
aiming for.

Set specific goals. Lose weight for a positive reason – it's good for your health, you want to live longer, you want more energy, not just because you 'need to lose weight'.

Think long term. You are making these changes to improve your life. You are working towards being the person you want to be forever, not just looking for a quick fix.

Do it for a bet. Set an affordable amount and wager that you can win. This works well if you are proud and competitive!

Do it for charity. The celebrities who took part in *Fit Club* each made a donation to a favourite charity. Losing weight for someone else, especially a good cause, and being sponsored to do it can be very motivating.

Do it for your children. They deserve and need to have you around for a long time, and being over-weight means that you are putting your health and life-expectancy at risk.

Give yourself rewards that are not food-linked. You should congratulate yourself when you have done well, but try not to see this in terms of, 'I deserve a bar of chocolate'. At the end of a week of weightloss and sustained exercise, promise yourself an evening out at the movies, a new dress, a new pair of jeans, even just a new pair of underpants! Eventually your new way of life will become second nature and you won't need rewards for behaviour that has become the norm.

Keep busy. If you are bored you will be far more tempted to reach for a bag of crisps or a packet of biscuits. When you feel tempted, especially at those low points of the day (mid-morning, late afternoon), find yourself something to do – preferably something physical like walking around the office, walking down to the Post Office, or weeding the garden.

Try not to get hungry. See Chapter 4 on avoiding hunger pangs.

Be aware of bad habit triggers. Do you find your-self buying a bar of chocolate when you buy the news-paper or fill up with petrol? Do you shop on the way home from work when you are hungry? Avoid the times when you are most likely to give in to tempta-tion by trying to change the way you do things. Go to a different shop, or at a different time of day when you are less hungry. People who eat in front of the TV also eat more. Endeavour to eat at the table. Break those habits!

Eat more slowly and savour the taste. It's very easy to bolt down food without really enjoying it, and it's a sure-fire way of eating more than you should. Appreciate each mouthful and less may be enough.

Talk to yourself. Not as mad as it sounds. Looking at yourself in the mirror and saying aloud, 'I will lose weight', 'I am doing well' can be surprisingly motivating.

Use a tape measure. Take a note of your measurements before you start your new healthy lifestyle and keep a weekly record, ideally on a graph, so that you can really see for yourself how much fat you have lost. Use the charts on pages 210-211.

Keep a weight chart and fill it in every week to prove to yourself that the trend is downward.

Play to your strengths. If you are an organized person and like to be businesslike, approach your weightloss and exercise as you would a business plan. Make lists, set goals, create a spreadsheet. Are you a good cook? Experiment with a whole new way of cooking with healthier options (see Chapter 8 for some recipes from Champneys chef, Adam Palmer). Are you a morning person? Get up a little earlier and start your day with thirty minutes' exercise.

Choose a person you want to impress. For extra motivation, select your partner/doctor/best friend/ mother – someone whose approval is important to you – and aim to amaze them.

Start the changes in yourself now. Why not try a new hairstyle, buy a different pair of spectacles, experiment with make-up. Find easy ways to begin to change which will make you feel different and good about yourself.

Look at other areas of your life. By losing weight and getting fit, you are on the way to a new you. There may be other areas of your life you are unhappy with – your job, the mess in your house, your relationships – which may even be contributing to your eating habits. Ask yourself if you can do something to improve these situations.

Find a photograph of yourself when slimmer and stick it on the fridge. Each time you open the fridge, say to yourself, 'That's the way I want to be again'.

Feel that weight: Each week put into a backpack things that weigh the amount you have lost – this could be in the form of tins of beans, bags of sugar, books – then put it on your back to show yourself graphically just how much weight you have lost.

Clear out your wardrobes, cupboards and drawers of clothes that fit you now and take them to the charity shop. Then there is no going back. You will need new clothes, but in a smaller size...

Keep one souvenir of your fat days and bring it out every now and then to reaffirm your success.

Keep a visual diary of your changing shape. Have photos taken of you monthly, and keep them in a box under your bed. Take them out when you are feeling low and see how your shape has changed.

Say a mantra. Choose a sentence to repeat to yourself

to reaffirm your ambition. 'I will be slimmer', 'I have a small appetite', 'I will go out for a walk/jog today'.

Avoid negative feelings. This is not a punishment. The classic failed dieters' excuse is to say, 'I lost the weight but it went back on *when I started eating again*'. This makes a change in your food habits sound like deprivation. How awful to imagine that you can't have pastry/a pork pie/a piece of chocolate ever again! This is where crash diets fail – they do not work around a realistic lifestyle: we are all human. Think in terms of an overall change of habit.

Don't use the 'D' word. By its very nature, a diet sounds temporary. You are not on a diet, you are changing the way you eat *forever*.

Try to express the changes in your life in positive terms. Rather than saying, 'I don't eat chocolate much anymore'; announce: 'I eat yogurts and fruit for pudding now'.

Avoid can'ts. Try not to say, 'I can't diet'; better to think, 'I can eat better'.

Avoid excuses. Are you hearing yourself say, 'I can't go for a walk – it's raining', 'I haven't time for any exercise today', 'There's no point in bothering to eat better tonight, we're going out to dinner'? So? Take an umbrella; get up earlier or use your lunch break; drink plenty of water before dinner and choose the healthier options from the menu.

Tell people what you are doing. Many will be surprisingly supportive and it will boost your confidence if people comment on how good you look each time they see you, but...

Be selective about who you tell. If the world and his wife know you are trying to lose weight, there will be some people who will appoint themselves the voice of your conscience ('Should you be eating that?'). This will make you resentful and more inclined to give in and say, 'What the heck' and eat another slice of pizza just to be contrary!

Don't let people bully you. They may have their own agenda for wanting you to join them in a cream cake. People who are failing to lose weight – especially those on the type of diets that promise spectacular results in a month – will be jealous of you and may try to undermine your success.

Steer clear of failed 'dieters'. You may be one yourself, but this is about a lifechange, not a thirty-days-to-the-perfect body temporary diet. People will relish telling you, 'It won't work' just because some diet they have tried didn't work for them.

Give in perhaps, but never give up.

Don't weigh yourself more than once a week. Your weight can fluctuate from day to day – water retention being one reason. It is counterproductive even if the general trend is downward. To see that you have put on a few ounces can be very demotivating.

Be patient! We live in a society where we want everything to happen now! But weight loss that is sustainable and permanent has to happen slowly and steadily, and physical changes may not happen straightaway, especially if you have a lot to lose. Aim for 1kg of weightloss each week (that's more than a stone in two months), and suddenly people will begin to notice.

Don't be put off by bad days. One day when you slip into old habits does no harm. You can regroup and make tomorrow better. You are only one meal away from getting back on track.

Be kind to yourself. Forgive yourself if you have eaten something you shouldn't have or have taken the car when you could have walked. It's not the end of the world. There is always tomorrow to get back on track. Most of all forgive yourself for having become overweight and inactive. That's in the past. Look to the future.

You make decisions about your life and your family all the time. You probably make decisions at work for the benefit of the company, your clients or customers. You may have children and need to take very seriously their education and welfare. You no doubt have to consider carefully the best way to handle your money/insurance/mortgage.

Now is the time to make decisions about yourself and your health and take them just as seriously. You are the most important project you will ever have to handle. Make it your best decision yet!

CHAPTER 4

THE WAY TO EAT

We hope you've got the message now that the way to successful and lasting weightloss is through exercise and a healthy eating regime. But what *is* healthy eating? Dr Adam Carey, our nutrition expert, is convinced that hitting the right balance is the secret to achieving a healthy weight – no more cutting out food types or dramatically reducing your calories. But to find the right balance it helps to understand food and the effect it has on our bodies. There's more to a meal than satisfying your appetite. Here's how to make food work for you.

How food turns to fat
If you've been tucking into takeaways and chomping chocolate with abandon, you'll know why you've piled on the pounds. But what if you have been careful about what you eat, dutifully following all the expert advice on healthy eating, and find that you are still putting on weight? You've gone for carbohydrates in your diet and cut out the fat, just like they told you to. What's gone wrong? It's just not fair! But, actually, it may not be your fault after all!

The latest research on diet and weightgain shows that this high-carb/low-fat style of eating is not as good for us than we once thought, and once you understand the way your body works, it's easy to see why. When we eat food that is highly processed and rich in carbohydrates – like white bread, sugary cereal (including many low-fat options which often have additional sugar added to them), pasta, cakes and biscuits, rice and potatoes – the food is digested quickly and easily and is then converted into glucose that is released into our blood to provide energy for our cells.

Everyone, fat or thin, should cut down on the refined, sugar-laden diet so common in the UK, but high-energy intake is fine when you're young or if you are very active, which is why most energetic teenagers manage to eat what they like and still stay skinny. They burn up the glucose provided by carbohydrates to create the energy they need. But so many of us lead sedentary lives nowadays that this process just doesn't happen and, if we don't modify our diet, our bodies can no longer deal with what we eat. The sudden rise in blood glucose levels triggers the release of insulin, a hormone produced by the pancreas. Insulin helps glucose to be burnt as energy in the cells, and turns some of it into glycogen, a readily available form of energy stored in the muscles and liver, but when there is more glucose than we need, and we are not burning it off, insulin is responsible for it being turned into fat. By consistently eating more carbohydrates than we can use, we stimulate the production of insulin and end up storing fat.

It gets worse. Insulin also plays a part in appetite. It can warn your brain that you are getting hungry and need to top up your energy levels. The trouble is that the high levels of insulin we are producing in response to our Western, high-carb diet means that we are feeling hungry soon after eating. This kind of high-carb food is everywhere – we're surrounded by snack and fast foods! And it's easy to see why. They are cheap to produce, easy to transport and store, quick to eat – even when you're on the move – and give a quick (if very temporary) feeling of satisfaction. So we eat more, produce more insulin, store what we've just eaten as fat...then feel hungry again. And so it goes on in a vicious circle.

Why dieting makes you fat

All the members of *Celebrity Fit Club* had tried dieting in the past – with the usual results. Despite losing weight initially, they had all found it impossible to keep it off. As their weight loss slowed, they felt less like sticking to their restrictive and punishing diets, and eventually went back to their previous style of eating and they regained most, if not all, of the weight they had lost. In some cases, they had actually ended up being heavier than before they started. Many people have had the same experience.

Adam Carey was able to explain why this was and, in doing so, went a long way towards dispelling the tremendous sense of failure that results from repeated, unsuccessful dieting. 'The whole point of faddy, crash diets is to get you to eat less calories, a lot less calories. As a consequence of this, you do lose weight. But the weight you lose is predominantly muscle mass. And as you lose your muscle mass what you notice is that you become weaker and have less energy. And with this your basic metabolic rate (BMR) – the rate at which your cells turn over energy when you're at rest – is reduced.'

Adam explained that your body is like a car. 'If you

have got a car with a three-litre engine, even if you just leave the engine running without going anywhere, it uses an awful lot of petrol, but if you have a moped with a 50cc engine, the same amount of petrol will last three, four, five, even ten times as long. When you crash diet or when you use a fad diet, it's as if you reduce the size of the engine you have inside you. And so you need fewer calories even to keep it ticking over.

'When you stop that diet – and everybody stops dieting at some stage – and go back to eating as you did before, then two things happen. Firstly you're eating the same number of calories as you were before but now you've got a smaller engine, so those additional calories get converted into body fat. Secondly, your body is desperate to try and repair itself because obviously this crash-dieting has caused a lot of damage to it, so it starts to rebuild its engine, it rebuilds your muscle mass. And while it does that, it tucks away a little bit of extra fat to protect you just in case you should be subjected to such a terrible siege again. It lays down extra supplies for next time.'

So now we know that our traditional Western eating habits are making us fat, but that diets don't work. Where does that leave us?

The Plan
To end your weight problems for good, you're going to have to rethink:
• How you eat
• What you eat
• How much you eat
• When you eat

This might sound a bit daunting, but the chances are that you don't really like the way you eat at the moment – and you certainly don't like the way it makes you feel. So what have you got to lose? You know exactly what (and how much), so let's get going.

How you eat: enjoying your food

When you've been battling with your weight for years, it's easy to start regarding food as the enemy. But it doesn't have to be that way. Adam feels strongly that, as a nation, we've forgotten how to eat and that we don't truly appreciate our food any more. With Adam's eating plan, you'll organize yourself to eat appetizing, good quality food when you need it, rather than feeling that you're starving yourself for most of the day. This is food you can enjoy.

Many of us have developed habits based around food and drink – doughnuts bought on the way to work, tea and biscuits in the afternoon, a couple of pints or a glass of wine with a bag of crisps after work – and these all contribute to the imbalances in our daily food intake. Thinking about these habits and finding ways to avoid them or to divert ourselves from them is all part of the strategy. Many of us have been overeating for so long that we no longer recognize the signs of real hunger or of satisfaction when we have eaten. By making small changes to our diets and habits, we can go a long way towards rediscovering our natural, healthy appetites.

Here are some tips to help you break your bad eating habits and form new, more positive ones:

Make meals you can really enjoy. To maintain a programme of healthy eating that will provide you with all the energy you need, and help you stay at a steady, healthy weight you can select ingredients from the lists in this chapter and combine them to suit you. This will take organization and forward planning, but the results are certainly worth it.

Give your appetite a chance to be heard again! When you are about to reach for some food, stop and think about just how hungry you are. Rate your hunger as a percentage. If you're tempted to snack at around 20 or 30 per cent, then something other than hunger is driving you. See below for suggestions on how to cope with grazing habits. Eat at around 60 per cent of your hunger, but be careful not to leave it until you reach 80 per cent or over. If you remember to eat one of Adam's protein/carbohydrate snacks (see pages 105-106) between your main meals, you should never be ravenous.

Before you eat anything, stop and really look at it. Take a moment to consider if it really is the best choice for you at that moment. How will it make you feel if you eat it? How will you feel in half and hour, or in two hours? Sometimes taking a moment to think will be enough to help guide you to a better selection of food.

Slow down when you eat. Give your brain a chance to catch up with your stomach so it will know when you've eaten enough. Pay attention to how you feel as you eat, and when you feel satisfied. Chew each mouthful carefully, take smaller mouthfuls, put your knife and fork down in between and pay attention to every bite, noticing and relishing all the flavours and textures.

Pay attention to your food and, when you're eating, make sure that it is your central activity. You're much more likely to ignore the signals that indicate you've eaten enough if you're distracted by television, listening to music or by chatting. Take care not to snack unconsciously at the fridge door, or pick at food as you cook a meal.

Use a smaller plate than usual. You can always take extra if you're still hungry, but the temptation to clear a big plateful, even when you're no longer hungry, is removed. If you can't bear to leave food on your plate, at least this way you won't be overeating. Try removing the serving dishes from the dining table once everyone has taken what they want. It's so tempting to pick at food that's right in front of you. If the dishes are in another room, you'll have to make a conscious effort to take more.

What you eat:
If your current eating habits are typical, you probably get:
• about 75 per cent of your daily calories from carbs
• 20-22 per cent from fat (mainly saturates)
• only about 5 per cent from protein.

Adam's plan involves changing this balance to:
- about 55 per cent carbs
- 30 per cent protein
- 15 per cent fat (mainly essential fats)

(See the following pages for types of foods in these groups.)
Although you'll be cutting down on refined carbs, you'll actually be eating more protein, including some of the foods you may have been avoiding for years, like lean meat, eggs and nuts. In addition, it's very important to keep eating small amounts of protein in the form of snacks between meals, so that you don't experience energy drops and cravings the way you probably do now. As for your choice of foods, we've made it easy by listing the foods that will give most benefit during your weightloss phase, but it will also be helpful if you understand a bit more about what you eat, and what it does for you.

Eat a balanced diet

Choose a wide variety of natural, unprocessed foods from all the food groups. These include carbohydrates (including vegetables, wholegrains and fruit), protein and fats.

By including a variety of foods in the diet, you increase the likelihood of consuming all the nutrients, vitamins and minerals that you require for a healthy and balanced diet. A variety of foods also ensures that your diet remains interesting and exciting.

Use cookbooks and try new recipes (like those in Chapter 8) to bring creativity and new tastes and flavours into your diet.

The right carbs

We're not suggesting that you should cut carbohydrates right out of your diet. You need them for energy, and, as Adam explained, not eating them at all would give you an unbalanced, faddy diet that could lead to health problems. It is far better to choose your carbohydrates with care, and to adjust how much you eat depending on whether you are trying to lose or maintain weight.

We now understand that carbohydrates are released into the blood as glucose at different rates. For many foods this has been measured and given a rating called the *Glycaemic Index* (GI). Foods with a high GI lead to a fast increase in blood glucose, resulting in a tremendous surge in insulin production. Foods with a low GI release their energy over a longer period. These are the ones to choose if you want to beat sugar cravings because they satisfy your appetite and provide energy over a longer period. You will find a list of carbohydrate foods with their GI on pages 111-113.

• Most people get about 75 per cent of their energy from carbohydrates. Try to reduce this to about 50 per cent.

• Wholegrains and fibrous vegetables are a good choice of carbohydrate.

• Avoid refined carbohydrates such as white rice, white flour products and processed breakfast cereals.

• Foods that taste sweet (biscuits, cakes and sweets) are absorbed quickly, have high glycaemic indices and offer no vitamins and minerals.

Fibre

Some of the more extreme low-carb diets can result in constipation, because fibre is found in unrefined carbohydrate foods such as whole grains, vegetables and fruit. Cutting these out means that you cut out the fibre too – with uncomfortable results. The plan Adam recommends reduces carbohydrates somewhat, but maintains a healthy intake of high-fibre vegetables.

There are two types of fibre: soluble and insoluble. Insoluble fibre has a bulking effect, whereas soluble fibre is inclined to form gel, retaining water in the bowel and keeping stools soft. This sort of insoluble fibre is found in oats, vegetables, wholewheat flour, bran, and fruits with edible seeds. Soluble fibre is found in oats, pulses, barley, bananas, apples, pears, citrus fruits, berries. Both types should be included in a healthy diet.

Fibre has been identified as having many other beneficial effects including control of blood glucose, decreasing blood cholesterol, improving bowel health and even controlling appetite. It also slows the rate of digestion and absorption of nutrients, thus reducing swings in blood sugar control.

On average, we consume between 10 to 20g of dietary fibre a day. Ideally we should consume at least 30 to 40g per day.

If you think your fibre intake needs some serious attention, increase your intake gradually each day.

Make sure you are well hydrated as fibre retains water in the bowel.

Fruit and vegetables

While you are in your weightloss phase, do not replace all your servings of vegetables with fruit, some types of which have a high glycaemic index. Aim for four to five servings of vegetables each day and one to two portions of fruit.

Vegetables that grow above the ground (i.e. cabbage, broccoli, spinach, rhubarb, beans and peas) have a high dietary fibre content and contain antioxidants and phytochemicals that help reduce the risk of heart disease and many cancers.

Balance your vegetable intake between the orange/red and green varieties. The more colourful the meal, the healthier it usually is and, as an easy rule, the darker and brighter the colour of the vegetable the more vitamins, minerals and fibre it will contain.

Vegetables can be eaten raw and cooking most of them takes only a few minutes if you steam, stir-fry or microwave them.

Protein power – or defeating those hunger pangs

One of the things that worried the members of *Fit Club* is something that will be familiar to anyone who has tried to lose weight – the fear of feeling hungry. That sense of deprivation is particularly dangerous, because it can result in your feeling so hard done by that you binge on unhealthy foods, just to regain a feeling of being full. Also, many people simply enjoy eating, and worry that they won't be able to relish their food in the way they usually do because their food will be unappetizing. This doesn't happen with Adam Carey's eating plan.

Meals and snacks based round refined carbohydrates provide a feeling of fullness, which doesn't last and very soon afterwards you could eat the whole thing over again. This is something we've all experienced: eating a couple of biscuits, then drifting back for a few more. And before you know it, half the pack has gone.

But there are foods that will provide lasting satisfaction, and that will take you effortlessly to your next meal without your having to experience hunger pangs. The magic formula is to base your meals around protein together with some complex carbohydrates. So if you have a piece of fish and some salad for lunch it'll see you through to your afternoon snack very comfortably. But if you've just had a baguette, then about an hour later you could have a little bar of chocolate or some other refined carbohydrate snack – and the whole cycle starts again.

Promoting protein

Most people get only about 5 per cent of their daily energy from protein. Try to increase this to at least 20–25 per cent.

Eat some protein at every meal and in your snacks. Protein helps to control blood glucose levels, supports muscle and therefore your metabolic rate, and improves appetite control.

Choose from a wide variety of protein sources. See the next page for a list of protein-rich foods that are both appetizing and healthy.

Protein pick list

• Eggs are rich in nutrients, cheap and a high quality source of protein.

• Choose lean meat and poultry.

• Avoid prepared meals and processed meats like pâté, salami and sausages.

• Fish is a superb source of protein; it is low in fat and some fish has the added advantage of being high in omega-3 fatty acids. Avoid deep-fried fish products that have been coated and battered. In your weightloss phase, use tinned fish in mineral water rather than oil.

• Grill, bake, steam or poach fish instead of frying.

• Avoid pork, as it is the most fatty of red meats.

• Peas and beans (legumes) are excellent sources of protein and fibre, especially when combined with wholegrains.

Most plant proteins do not contain all the essential amino acids, which are the building blocks of proteins (animal protein does); combining different sources of plant protein solves this problem. Legumes should be eaten with wholegrains, e.g. brown rice and lentils, houmous with wholewheat pitta bread.

Plant proteins are very low in fat and have a very low glycaemic index (see page 111), which means that they cause a slow release of glucose into the blood. Baked beans have a low glycaemic index, are cheap, convenient and easy to store.

Nuts are also a useful protein source but they should be eaten in moderation as they have a high essential fat content. Choose a mixture of almonds, pecans, walnuts, and Brazil nuts, hazelnuts, cashews, pumpkin, sunflower and sesame seeds. Add them to a salad or stir-fry, or eat them as a snack. Avoid salted nuts and those that have been roasted in oil.

Soya milk and soya yogurt can work well as dairy substitutes. Eating soya products may reduce the incidence of a number of diseases including breast cancer, osteoporosis, heart disease and prostate cancer in men. Women with endometriosis (a uterine abnormality) should limit their intake of soya.

Drink up!

It's very important to make sure that your body has enough water at all times. Being properly hydrated is essential to your health, and even a small loss of water can lead to both your mind and your body operating below par.

• The average adult needs to drink at least 2-3 litres of water a day, and more if you exercise.

• Don't put off drinking until you feel thirsty. Thirst is a poor measure of dehydration. You become dehydrated long before you feel thirsty so drink water continuously throughout the day. Being well hydrated improves how you feel and perform.

• Alternatively, choose fruit teas and herbal blends, and water flavoured with a little fresh fruit juice.

• The best measure of fluid balance is urine colour; this should be clear and pale at all times. Dark yellow urine is an indicator of dehydration. Some multivitamins may give the urine a bright yellow appearance.

• Caffeine is found in tea, coffee, chocolate and colas. Caffeine is a stimulant, increasing heart rate and blood pressure. It also irritates the stomach and can cause headaches and insomnia. A person who drinks more than eight cups of coffee a day would fail a drug test by the International Olympic Committee. Choose alternatives such as herb and fruit teas, fruit juice and water (still the best choice).

Booze and weightloss

Alcohol is very high in calories, it causes low blood sugar and dehydration. National guidelines suggest women should not exceed 14 units per week (21 for men). The less you drink, the healthier you are. A glass of red wine a day may have some health benefits but these benefits can easily be achieved elsewhere.

If it is socially difficult for you to avoid drinking at business lunches, alternate your drinks with a mineral water or dilute your drinks with soda or water.

WATER TRICKS

- Have filtered water at home and remember to use it to fill the kettle and for cooking.
- Start the day with a mug of freshly boiled water and a slice of lemon. In summer add a fresh sprig of mint and fresh lemon slices to a jug of cold water.
- Drink from a bottle of water to measure daily intake until you are used to drinking enough.
- Weigh yourself before and after exercise. For every kilogram lost, a litre of water is lost.

Good and bad fats

Contrary to popular belief, not all fats are bad, many are good and a *zero* fat or a very low-fat diet is harmful to your health in the long term.

• Saturated animal fats can increase the risk of heart disease, some cancers and stroke. Saturated fats are generally solid at room temperature. They are found in meat and dairy products – butter, cheese, for example.

• Other 'good' fats (containing the Omega-3 and Omega-6 essential fatty acids) are crucial to many functions of your body. They maintain skin and hair, they store and transport vitamins A, D, E and K, and support your immune system.

• You can't make these 'essential' fats in your body, so you have to eat them regularly. Omega-3 fatty acids are found in oily fish like salmon, trout, sardines, mackerel, herring and tuna – also great sources of protein. Try to eat this kind of fish around four times a week.

• Use only *cold pressed* vegetable oils such as virgin olive oil and flaxseed oil. These should be used for salads and not for cooking.

• For bread and toast, a small amount of butter is actually better than margarine, apart from the new brands that are advertised as lowering blood cholesterol as part of a good diet.

• Avoid frying and roasting foods and try to steam, grill and bake instead.

• For fat use an amount equivalent to the size of your thumb and try not to eat more fat than that at each meal (for most people that is somewhere between a dessert and tablespoonful of olive oil or the equivalent 'healthy fat').

How much to eat

Since this is not a diet, no food is banned and you do not have to count calories – just think about what you are eating and what it is doing for you. As you get your cravings under control by eating regular amounts of protein and by reducing high GI carbs, you'll be more aware of your appetite and will almost certainly find yourself eating less as a result. To help you get started you need a quick and simple way to assess how much you should be eating. Take a look at your hands!

Think of portions in relation to the size of the palm of your hand, minus the fingers and thumb, and about the same thickness.

• Each meal should contain protein. Eat between one and two palms-worth for main meals and half this amount for snacks, depending on how active you are throughout the day.

• For vegetables and salad, go for at least two palms for each main meal.

• Try not to eat more than one palm of starchy carbs at one sitting.

• For the amount of fat you should be eating at each meal, don't exceed an amount that would correspond to the volume of your thumb.

When to eat

All the members of *Celebrity Fit Club* wanted to reduce the amount of fat stored by their bodies, and that's a priority for most people starting a fitness regime. Adam had some useful advice for optimising fat-burning that would help celebrities achieve their goal more rapidly. 'If you can do the fat-burning part of your exercise first thing in the morning on an empty stomach, you'll actually burn a lot of fat calories. If you exercise at other times of the day you'll burn the same number of calories but they won't have come necessarily so much from body fat. So try to ensure that some of the fat-burning exercise (see page 122) you do in a week is done first thing in the morning on an empty stomach.'

Although unrefined carbohydrates form an important part of Adam's eating plan, he is not suggesting that we give up refined carbohydrates altogether. It's a question of reallocating them to the best time of day for our bodies. Fitting food together with exercise gives us the best chance of providing our bodies with the fuel they need to function at their best. Refined carbs, like pasta, bread or rice are great to eat after you've exercised. So if you've gone to the gym on the way home from work, or done your exercise in the early part of the evening, then your evening meal at six-thirty or seven o'clock is the ideal time to have a bowl of pasta, because it actually tops up the stores of sugar in muscle and liver that have been depleted through exercise. But think in terms of using refined carbs to top up after exercise, rather than exercising to work off refined carbs you've given in to!

If you need any more encouragement to start exercising regularly, just read what Adam has to say about exercise and appetite: 'Exercise seems to reduce your appetite so it has a very positive effect on appetite. As you start to exercise these things start to feed into one another and they start to self-support. Exercise and diet go together hand in hand. If you do one without the other, most of the time you'll make short-term progress but you won't make long-term progress. And when you exercise first thing in the morning, it sets up your metabolic rate for the whole day and makes it go that little bit faster. So it means that all day you burn slightly more calories.'

• Eat 'breakfast like a king, lunch like a prince and dine like a pauper', adding in two snacks for a well-balanced day.

• Skipping some meals and eating only one or two large meals a day results in poor energy levels, poor appetite control, muscle loss and uncontrolled blood glucose.

• Eating five smaller meals each day and including protein in each of them helps to control hunger levels, moods, and blood glucose levels and assists in preventing long-term fat storage.

Try to eat your last meal before 8pm. Going to bed while digesting your dinner is a poor recipe for a good night's sleep and encourages the conversion of calories into body fat.

CARBOHYDRATE HINTS

1. Replace some starchy carbs with fibrous carbs at each meal. This will increase fibre and help fill you up.
2. Avoid large carbohydrate meals, as these will make you sleepy, and excess calories will be converted into body fat.
3. Always choose wholegrain options. Brown rice, wholewheat cereal and wholegrain breads are always higher in nutrients and have a lower glycaemic index.
4. Starchy carbohydrates should be limited in the evening meal, as the need for an energy source at night is limited.

A weightloss regime for you

Adam has offered us 'go-faster stripes' to help us lose fat quickly while remaining healthy and energetic.

• Eat five to six evenly spaced meals, three main meals and two to three snacks.

• If you are hungry then eat more salad, vegetables and protein, rather than more starchy and fat-laden foods.

• Try to eat starchy carbohydrates earlier in the day (at breakfast) or directly following exercise.

• Choose these carbohydrates carefully. Use the glycaemic index (see page 111), choosing food with a low and medium glycaemic index rating for the most part, and include higher-rated foods only as rewards for exercise and activity.

• Don't try to cheat by using exercise to compensate for over-eating starchy carbs.

Remember that for the purposes of body fat reduction, fruit is classed as a starchy carb, and fruit juice is just refined fruit. Temperate fruits, like apples, pears, plums and berries are far preferable to tropical fruits like bananas, mangoes, peaches and grapes.

• Keep a diet and training diary.

• Snack on healthy foods – cut out the sweets and biscuits.

• Plan your meals and shop to provide for them.

• Expect to be uncomfortable at first with some of the changes you are making. This is only human nature. After all, you are stepping outside your comfort zone, and your new regime is going to take some getting used to.

• If you slip up, remember that you are only ever one meal away from getting back on track.

• Drink more water.

High-energy meals to take you through the day

Never skip **breakfast**! Base it around protein + starch:

Try:

Grilled bacon or other lean meat

Tomatoes and poached eggs on rye bread

Porridge, nuts and seeds

Eggs any style: scrambled with smoked salmon,
Spanish omelette, poached, boiled on
wholemeal toast

Sardines or baked beans on rye bread

Lunch: Protein + fibrous starch/proteins

Try:

Salads, such as salade Niçoise

Caesar salad or mixed bean and tuna salad

Greek salad with feta cheese, turkey, chicken or
cold salmon salads

Soup made from beans or pulses, or vegetable soup.
Add some form of protein like chopped-up
chicken breast or extra prawns

Dinner: Protein + fibrous starches + 'good fats'

Try:

Lots of vegetables. Be creative in ringing the
changes by roasting, grilling, steaming and
eating raw in salads

Stir-fried lean meats and vegetables minus the
rice and the noodles

Choose a good quality protein source (or two)
and make this the focus of your meal

Adapt meals like spaghetti bolognaise, by serving the sauce (made with lean meat) on a bed of red cabbage or broccoli instead of spaghetti

Snacks to get you though the day

With Adam's eating plan, no one should ever feel hungry. He has plenty of suggestions for healthy snacks that should definitely keep hunger pangs at bay, and avoid the kind of binge-eating that is so depressingly familiar to dieters. In addition to the three main meals of breakfast, lunch and dinner, Adam suggests two or three carefully planned snacks based around protein combined with complex carbohydrates to ensure long-lasting satisfaction.

This should prove ideal for Ann Widdecombe, whose erratic eating habits are a product of her packed schedule. Like so many people, who sit at their desks working, food is the last thing on her mind, but having to attend formal lunches throws temptation in her way on a regular basis. If she has not eaten during the morning, she is bound to feel hungry by lunchtime, and if she feels that she cannot allow herself to enjoy the food being served, the seeds are sown for her abandoning her eating plan and giving up the fight.

Six almonds and an apple: provide protein and some complex carbohydrate.

Two handfuls of raw vegetables: dip carrots, celery, pepper, mushrooms or courgettes in one tablespoon of cottage cheese, houmous or salsa. Raw vegetables are a healthy snack because they are high in complex carbohydrates and antioxidants, the naturally occurring compounds that help protect the body from disease.

A handful of nuts: packed with protein and minerals like selenium, zinc and magnesium, nuts provide essential nutrients that women tend to skimp on in their diets. They also contain antioxidants, vitamin E and are low in carbohydrates. Just remember to limit your portion to a handful and steer clear of roasted and salted varieties.

Pumpkin or sunflower seeds: just a handful of these provides essential omega-3 fatty acids, one of the most important types of dietary oils that help maintain healthy cells and skin as well as brain functionality.

A 150g pot of low-fat bio yogurt (preferably organic): with some fruit stirred in, this is an excellent source of protein and rich in calcium, which helps to build strong bones.

Two oat cakes topped with cottage cheese, houmous, ham or turkey: a satisfying low-fat option packed with calcium.

Good restaurant choices

As a population we now spend about £26 billion a year on eating out and about £5 billion on takeaways. If you're spending your hard-earned cash, make sure what you choose is going to help you achieve your goal of permanent weightloss.

Adam's top tips for eating out

While you're trying to lose weight you probably need to follow a 95/5 per cent rule, so you need to get things right 95 per cent of the time, and keep your indulgences – or slip-ups – down to 5 per cent. In a week that's twenty out of twenty-one meals which need to be pretty spot on; that one meal would be a very good opportunity to go out to a restaurant and bend the rules a bit. If you get the other twenty meals right, you're still on track.

• When you get to the weight you want to be, you can then play an 80/20 per cent rule. That means three or four meals a week can be a little bit more relaxed, for example Sunday lunch plus another three meals a week, particularly if you maintain your regular routine of exercise. But you can still use your new understanding of how food works to make healthier choices than you would have done before.

• When you're going out for dinner in the evening, don't go feeling ravenously hungry or you will order the whole menu – plus pudding! Remember to eat your four previous meals and snacks during the day, particularly your mid- or late-afternoon snack.

• Another good way of curbing your appetite at dinner is to go to the gym or do your exercise in the evening just before going out, because this will reduce your appetite too.

• The first thing you should order is a bottle of water. Many people confuse hunger with thirst, so you may think you're very hungry when what your body is really saying to you is that you're very thirsty. Have a glass of water while you're looking at the menu.

• When making your choices from the menu, think starters and main courses, but don't even look at the desserts. If you're still genuinely hungry, you can order this later.

• Consider fish for your main course. Many people don't cook fish at home, so eating out gives you the opportunity to try something new and very healthy.

• When you're looking at side orders to go with the main courses, think about replacing the chips or jacket potato with a salad and vegetables.

• When you're considering the carbohydrates in the main course, make a choice of whether you want to eat them or drink them. If you're designated driver for the evening, you're not going to be drinking any alcohol at all, and you could order the jacket potato that comes with the main course. But on a night when you're not driving and you fancy two or three glasses of wine, then choose to drink the calories and have a side salad with the main course instead.

• Don't always assume that the vegetarian option will be healthier. In many restaurants, the veggie dishes are covered in cheese, a rich source of saturated fat.

• Watch out for the meals which are just loaded with carbohydrate, such as pasta, pizza or club sandwich with a big portion of chips on the side. These are definitely ones to avoid because there is very little protein in any of them and they're not very well-balanced main courses.

• If you're having trouble finding a meal on the menu that looks just right, ask the waiter if you can order something a bit different. For example, ask for your meat or fish to be chargrilled and served without sauce, or ask for a large side salad (with dressing on the side) instead of cooked the standard cooked vegetables.

Takeaways and fast-food choices

Despite your best efforts at preparation and planning ahead, there are always going to be occasions when you have to try to make a healthy food choice in a fast-food restaurant. This is going to challenge your ingenuity to the extreme – because fast food is all about refined carbs, the worst kinds of fat, and often not very much protein.

An average takeaway meal could total 2500-3000 calories and you might then drink another thousand calories in beer, wine or carbonated drinks on top of that. This takes the total number of calories up to 3000-4000. If you're the correct weight, you could maybe get away with this a couple of times a week, but if you do it one extra time a week, you'll be putting on a pound of fat every single week. You can see how easy it is to put on a few stones over the course of a year just by having one extra takeaway or one extra meal every week.

If you're on the 95/5 part of your eating plan, you'll have to cut right down on this kind of food – or take evasive action to rebalance the nutrients. If you've achieved your ideal weight, however, you can cut yourself some slack. But you may be surprised to find that what used to be your favourite takeaway no longer seems quite so enjoyable – and certainly doesn't make you feel good. Once you've re-educated your appetite, you'll find it easier to make the healthier choice – because you just won't fancy the alternative!

Chinese

Opt for black bean and oyster sauce rather than sweet and sour

Go for plain boiled rice as opposed to fried rice
Avoid deep-fried starters – choose soup instead
Order satays and grilled meat, but go easy on sauces

Indian

Choose drier meat curries like jalfrezi
Avoid creamy sauces or dishes that come topped
  with ghee (Indian refined butter).
Choose tandoori and tikka, rather than the
  tikka masala with its creamy sauce.
Choose boiled rice rather then pilau rice
Try vegetable dishes
Avoid deep-fried dishes
Don't order naan bread

Burger restaurants

Never order a milk shake
If you have food in a bread roll, like a burger or
  sandwich, discard one half of the bread at least or
  just eat the filling
Choose diet versions of soft drinks
Don't be tempted to upgrade to a larger size just
  because it's cheap. Be guided by your appetite.
Try to slow down the rate at which you eat, to give
  your appetite a chance to guide you.

Fish and chips

You might as well make this the 5 per cent part of your
95/5 per cent rule, because fish and chips without the
chips, and fish without the batter are just not worth
eating! Pickled egg, anyone?

Glycaemic Index (GI) – your guide to choosing the right carbs

Low – these should be your carbs of choice

Asparagus	
Broccoli	Chick peas (cooked)
Bean sprouts	Peaches
Cabbage	Carrots (raw)
Cauliflower	Figs (fresh)
Celery	Oranges
Cucumber	Pears
Garlic	Quinoa (cooked)
Green vegetables	Yogurt (full-milk)
Lettuce	Yogurt (skimmed)
Mushrooms	
Radishes	
Onions	
Red peppers	
Tomatoes	
Grapefruit	
Peanuts	
Cherries	

Dark chocolate (70% cocoa solids)
Lentils - Green and Brown
Peas - Split and Dried (cooked)
Plums
Apples
Beans - French
Beans - Haricot

Medium – eat in moderation
Aubergine
Pumpernickel bread
Kidney beans
Orange juice (freshly squeezed)
Peas (fresh petits pois)
Rye (wholemeal bread)
Bulgar (wholegrain, cooked)
Pasta (durum wheat, cooked al dente)
Wholemeal bread
Kiwi fruit
Rice – Basmati and Brown
Sweet potato

High – avoid these carbs or eat in very small quantities, along with carbs with a low GI

Biscuits
Crackers
Rice (Long grain, White)
Bananas
Brown bread
Jam
Marmalade
Melon
Orange juice (from concentrate)
Potatoes (boiled in their skins or peeled and boiled)
Raisins
Cereals (sugared)
Chocolate bars (e.g. Mars Bar)
Soft drinks
Cornflour
Granary bread
Sugar
Turnips
Pumpkin
Watermelon
Broad beans (cooked)
Potato crisps
Tapioca
Carrots (cooked)
Cornflakes
Baguettes
Popcorn (no sugar)
Honey
Mashed potato

CHAPTER 5

THE WAY TO EXERCISE

What is exercise? Basically it is any increase in activity that gets your heart beating faster. Sadly it has very negative connotations in people's minds. It usually comes wrapped in sentences like, 'I must take some exercise' as if it were a form of punishment, or it conjures up images of super-fit, super-lean bodies pumping iron and pounding the treadmill in some overpriced gym. The former perception is demotivating. The latter is terrifying and boring!

But although exercise is an essential part of achieving a healthy body and successful weightloss, it really doesn't have to be like that. The secret is to find the kind of exercise that suits you and that fits into your life. Exercise can be very stimulating, and almost habit-forming, and once you feel yourself getting fitter, *not* exercising will become abnormal. You'll find something is missing from your day. Honest!

Finding the exercise that suits you

You'll know from completing your personal profile in Chapter 2 what kind of person you are. You might be allergic to gyms, have a sedentary or very stressful job with long hours; you may prefer to exercise alone or need to be with other people. You may even hate exercise – or at least activities you have tried in the past. Be prepared to juggle the hours in the day, and keep an open mind about the variety of exercise options available to you. Choose an activity which appeals and which fits in with your attitudes and your time.

• If you are at home in the daytime, set aside a few minutes at a particular time of the day when you can exercise. If you have children, ask a friend or neighbour to babysit for a while, or once your partner comes home, hand over the kids and grab some time for yourself before your evening meal.

• Work in an office? Take some time to exercise at the beginning of the day, or once you get home from work, before you sit down to eat or watch TV. Grab the opportunity to exercise whenever you can: get off the bus a stop early, or park your car a long way from the office and walk the rest of the way. Use your lunch hour to walk briskly for half an hour three times a week.

• Avoid the easiest option: take the stairs not the lift. Park your car in the space furthest away from the supermarket door.

• Look at ways to exercise at home. If you can afford one, invest in an exercise bike or some very basic equipment or improvise (see below). Work exercising at home around things you enjoy doing: watching TV, listening to music.

• Is there a spare room in your house – or corner of a room – that you can use as your 'gym'? It helps to be able to leave equipment out ready for use.

• If you need motivation, join a gym. It doesn't have to be an expensive one, but make sure that it is easy to get to, so that there are no obstacles in your way. You don't even need to buy full membership: many gyms offer cheaper memberships for restricted use of the facilities or for off-peak users.

• Join a local sports club or leisure centre (their membership rates are much cheaper than private gyms), and use the pool, knock around a football, play badminton, take part in a beginners' low-impact aerobics or step class. Don't be shy: everyone is there for the same reasons as you, and no one will be judgmental. If you had the body of an Adonis, you wouldn't be there!

• Are you competitive? Ask at your local sports club if they offer team sports you can become involved in.

• Find something you used to enjoy doing when you were younger – badminton, yoga, basketball. You may rediscover a dormant talent!

• Get – or borrow – a dog! Dogs have masses of energy and most breeds will walk for a long time. If there is a cycle track near you, take your bike and let the dog run alongside you.

Whatever you decide to do, do it whenever you can!

Avoid making excuses

Overweight people are good at making excuses. All the members of the *Fit Club* could find reasons to do no or very little exercise. They had filming schedules, an early start in the morning, or they got home too late. Once you are heavy, exercising is harder to do so it's a Catch 22 situation. But – as you saw in Chapter 1 – you need to be honest with yourself. As Harvey Walden said to the *Fit Club* members: 'My job is to assist and to guide you in changing your lifestyle. This will enable you to lose some weight, but the ultimate responsibility is on you. You must be part of the solution. Start off as a winner by not saying can't or never. Winners come up with solutions to problems not excuses.

Saying you don't have time is a poor excuse for not having a healthy life. It's not a chore, it's a lifestyle – your life and your health.'

Measuring fitness

You probably know how fit or unfit you are. You'll know by how it feels when you have to run for a bus or rush home in the rain. Do you get out of breath walking up the stairs, or can you walk briskly for ten or fifteen minutes before being out of breath? Work out your stamina by testing yourself with Harvey's assessment, then build up your exercise levels slowly:

• Run or walk/run very briskly for a quarter of a mile (you can measure a quarter of a mile on the mileometer in the car before you assess yourself).

• On the floor, ground or on a mat do 10 press-ups followed by 20 crunch curls (see pages 139-140).

• Completely out of breath and struggling? You need to build up your exercise slowly.

• Manageable? Set the intensity a little higher as it becomes easier.

How and why exercise works

Health and fitness experts get very technical about exercise – which is what puts lots of people off. It's actually not rocket science, but very simple and easy to work out.

Basically there are two sorts of exercise: anaerobic and aerobic. What's the difference?

Anaerobic Exercise (meaning without air) is intense – sprinting, running up the stairs, hurdling at the Olympics – when the heart is working at about 80-90 per cent of its maximum heart rate (MHR – see page 123). The heart cannot pump blood and oxygen to the muscles quickly enough during this type of exercise, so the body can only sustain it for about a minute. Even world class sprinters can only sustain this sort of intense exercise for a short time. Because the muscles have to work without oxygen (anaerobically), they burn carbohydrate. Lactic acid builds up in the muscles and the body is forced to ease off until enough oxygen gets to the muscles through the blood, so that the lactic acid can be recycled. This acid build-up explains the feeling of 'heavy legs' after intense activity.

Aerobic Exercise (with air) is a low-intensity form of exercise – walking briskly, light jogging, cycling – when the heart is able to pump oxygen around the body. It works at two intensity levels: cardiovascular training when the heart is beating at about 70-80 per cent of the maximum heart rate (see page 123), and lower intensity when the heart is beating at 60-70 per cent of the MHR. This is known as the *Fat-Burning Zone* – you may be breathing hard, but it's possible to sustain the exercise for longer. In this form of low-intensity exercise, the body starts by burning carbohydrates (glycogen stored in the muscles) for the first twenty minutes, and then starts to use fat stores to provide fuel. Keep the aerobic exercise at a low level and you will be able to sustain it for longer – perhaps half an hour to an hour – and, hey presto, you're burning fat!

How to keep aerobic exercise going

Half an hour to an hour's exercise isn't really that long – it could be a brisk walk during a TV programme you don't like, a hike down a country footpath, cycling to the shops on the other side of town, the duration of your favourite soap on the TV at the gym or at home.

• Make it fun or give yourself a purpose (to post a letter, buy the paper, walk the dog) and the time will pass quickly.

• If you are able to jog lightly for a while, that's great. Then ease off to a brisk walk to get your breath back and then jog again.

• Listen to some music. Put your favourite tape or CD on your Walkman as you exercise and make sure you keep going through a certain number of songs. (Be aware, though, that if you are walking or running near roads, you won't be able to hear approaching traffic with headphones on).

• Subscribe to exercise and fitness magazines. Harvey suggests you read them prior to a workout. Not only will they give you something to aim for – you will feel part of a community all doing the same thing as you.

When and how to exercise

Pick a time of day that suits you best – one where you have time to yourself so you aren't tempted to use the lack of it as an excuse to cut short your exercise time. Harvey suggests you plan your workouts as you plan everything else in your day. Make a note in your diary of what time you will set aside.

• Morning or later in the day? It entirely depends on you and your life. Exercise promotes energy though, so even if you are sluggish in the mornings now, you may find as you get fitter you have lots of energy at the beginning of the day.

• Exercise with a friend: you will help to spur each other on when one is feeling less enthusiastic. But make sure it's a friend who will motivate you – not one who will quit easily. You need support not diversion!

• Despite his incredibly fit body and a running regime that would make most people's hair curl, Harvey admits he does not particularly enjoy running. So what's his secret to getting motivated? 'I make sure I have trainers that are a joy to wear, or a new piece of kit. Something that makes me feel good.'

• Vary your exercises to avoid boredom. Anything becomes boring if you do it too often, so in a week cycle one day, swim another day, walk on the third.

• Keep a diary of your exercises and your times (you can use the chart on pages 214-215). It will help enormously to know as the weeks go by that you can run for longer, or cycle further; that you have increased the number of crunches or press-ups you can manage.

• Always warm up and cool down properly (see pages 134 and 139 for suitable ways to do this). This will help you to avoid injury. (See Chapter 7 for more tips).

Eating and exercise

It's not a good idea to exercise when you are feeling really hungry, but nor should you if you have just eaten. Because you are exercising to burn fat, leave a gap of at least an hour after you have eaten before you work out. When we eat, the pancreas releases the hormone insulin, which for a short time stops fat being used as a source of energy. Also blood is diverted to your stomach to help digestion after you have eaten, and this can leave you feeling lethargic and sleepy. You are also less likely to get a stitch.

Before or after breakfast? Adam Carey advises that it is better to exercise on an empty stomach. 'Some of the best times to burn off your calories in terms of fat-burning is first thing in the morning. The reason for that is that you can access your body fat as an energy source much more easily having not eaten anything, than after you've eaten. On an empty stomach, you'll actually burn a lot of fat calories.' If you need a boost, have one of the snacks recommended half an hour before you start to exercise.

When you have finished exercising
High-energy drinks are marketed vigorously as the 'essential equipment' for the athlete in replacing energy. But be wary of them. If they are low-calorie, they won't provide any energy at all. If they are not, they are glucose – i.e. pure sugar. Certainly energy does need to be replaced as you exercise (you need to replace the glycogen in your muscles), but these glucose drinks should be heavily diluted to make them only about 3-5 per cent glucose, and they should be drunk during the exercise session or immediately afterwards – especially if you can't face food after exercising. But the most important thing is to re-hydrate. Drink plenty of water during and after exercise.

Injury and when not to exercise
There are two types of pain when you exercise:
• One comes from using muscles that haven't been exercised for a long time. It is the weakness leaving

your body and the start of really effective exercise.

• The other is the pain you feel from overdoing it. You may not have warmed up properly and so have pulled a muscle. Overweight people often suffer from joint problems too. Stop when you feel this sort of injury pain, apply ice wrapped in a cloth to the muscle and support the muscle firmly but not too tightly.

• Overdoing exercise will inevitably lead to injury and could lay you up for weeks, undoing all the good you have done.

• Don't exercise if you feel unwell or have a fever.

• Always stop exercising *immediately* if you feel: dizzy, pain (especially in the chest) or faint.

Getting that heart working!

During exercise your heart rate increases to supply oxygen to the muscles and the harder you exercise, the faster your heart beats. This is the best way to burn fat. When you begin, exercise at least three times a week for a period of about 20-30 minutes: it's not until you have been going for 20 minutes that your body starts to use up fat reserves (see 'aerobic exercise' on page 118). The *Fat-Burning Zone* is the optimum heart rate for burning fat – the muscle cells are forced to derive most of their energy from fat reserves – but your heart is like any muscle: the fitter it is the more efficient it becomes at pumping the blood. As you get fitter, you will need to step up your exercise routine to reach the best level for burning fat.

Everyone has a maximum heart rate where, even if intensity were increased, the rate would remain the same.

Calculating your maximum heart rate
(220 minus your age):
18 years old: 220 - 18 = 202 BPM
25 years old: 220 – 25 = 195 BPM
30 years old: 220 – 30 = 190 BPM
40 years old: 220 – 40 = 180 BPM
55 years old: 220 – 55 = 165 BPM
BPM = beats per minute

As we said before, the rate that uses the greatest expenditure of energy consumption – or the best for fat burning – is at about 60-70 per cent of your maximum heart rate. By checking your beats per minute (BPM) as you exercise, you will discover how intensely and effectively you are working out. Once your heart is beating in the right zone, you are working at the right intensity.

Taking your BPM:
Take a few practice readings of your resting pulse, so you will be able to take an accurate reading once you are exercising.

1. Find your pulse (using your fingers not your thumb which has its own pulse) on the underside of your wrist or at the side of your neck under your jaw bone. You'll need to stop briefly if you are taking this reading whilst exercising.

2. Using the second hand of your watch, count the beats of your pulse for thirty seconds.

3. Multiply this figure by 2 and it will give you your heart rate per minute.

Doctors recommend that when you start exercising, you stay at the lower end (60 per cent) of your fat-burning zone. Once you become fitter, you can push it up to 85 per cent.

Age	Range for weight loss (beats/minute)
20	120-140
30	114-133
40	108-126
50	102-120
60	96-112

How much should you do to reach your Fat-Burning Zone? If you are very overweight, a brisk walk may be enough to get your heart pumping at the optimum rate. You'll discover as you exercise more and more, that you have to walk faster or for longer to maintain that rate. That's your body getting fitter. If the rate is too high (anaerobic exercise), you will exhaust yourself, and won't actually be burning any fat, so ease off.

IMPORTANT

Before you start exercising for the first time in ages, or if you are increasing the intensity of your exercise, Harvey stresses that you must get the green light from your doctor. 'He or she must also be aware of the type of exercise you are doing,' he says. 'and if your goal is to lose weight, tell him or her that you will be doing lots of cardiovascular exercise as this will raise your heart rate higher than light to moderate exercise.'

Get the kit!

Don't panic – we're not suggesting you dash down to the sports shop and bend your credit card on the latest designer outfits and equipment! You really don't need much in the way of equipment to exercise (so no excuses that it's too expensive): just a decent pair of trainers and barrels of determination. If you're the kind of person who likes to look the part though, that's fine. Sports equipment is designed to do its job properly, so moisture-wicking fabrics, cycling shorts, or branded jogging pants do the business and might make you feel that now you've got the kit, you had better put it to good use!

ESSENTIAL EQUIPMENT:

Training shoes: the design of these is now virtually a science and millions of pounds are invested by sportswear companies in research. Trainers need to give your feet the right support – after all, it's your feet that take the hammering. People unused to exercise, who may be heavy, should probably opt for motion-control shoes or stability shoes which are firm and durable. Cross trainers are designed to be suitable for most types of exercise. It is important to consider the shape of your feet when buying trainers: they may be normal, flat or high-arched (you can usually tell from the shape left by a wet footprint):

- Flat feet roll inwards – pronate
- High-arched feet roll outwards – supernate
- Normal feet are, well, normal! And stay virtually straight.

Take a look at your everyday shoes to see what shape they have formed into.

Where to buy them? The price range of trainers is truly mind-boggling, so take the advice of an expert from a sports shop (avoid cheap, chain store options). They can advise you on the correct ones for your feet and the type of exercise you plan to do. Try on several pairs before you decide, and don't fall for the most fashionable colour/style. You'll pay for the privilege.

A loose T-shirt, comfortable shorts or jogging pants and a sweatshirt for when it is cold are ideal for most sorts of exercise. Wear long sleeves for cycling, because even though you may work up a sweat, your arms can get cold in the wind.

A bike is a great idea, because cycling is an excellent form of exercise. You may have one gathering dust, so dig it out, pump up the tyres, oil the brakes and get pedalling. Make sure you wear a helmet and visible clothing. You'll need lights if you are planning to cycle in the dark. Sports shops sell bike stands which you can fix to your bike, enabling you to use it like an exercise bike.

A sturdy chair – a dining chair is ideal – as a support for strength-training exercises. (See page 140)

NON-ESSENTIAL EQUIPMENT:
A heart-rate monitor may be useful and was offered to all the *Fit Club* members. You strap a 'belt' around your chest when you exercise and the watch mechanism that you wear on your wrist gives you a reading of your BPM so you can check you are working within

your *Fat-Burning Zone*. These are cheap and available from most sports outlets.

A pedometer: Dr Chris Steele gave one of these to all the *Fit Club* members. It calculates how may steps you take in a day. The ideal amount is upwards of 10,000, and you'll be surprised how easy it is to achieve this number. Pedometers are not expensive and are available from most sports outlets. (See Chapter 10 for details on ordering both these items through mail order.)

A strong elastic band (you can buy special sports versions with varying resistance) is great for stretching and toning and resistance exercises. Make a loop in the middle for your foot and two loops at either end for handles to a length that means you have to pull it to reach.

Moisture-wicking running shirts are specially de- signed to wick away sweat as you exercise, and don't become heavy and wet, which is the downside of ordinary T-shirt material.

If your legs are big, **cycling shorts** will stop your thighs chafing together as you walk or run.

Handweights or dumb-bells are great for toning arms, but a couple of cans of baked beans will do the job just as well. When they become too light, increase the number of times you repeat the exercise or use a bag of flour or a couple of large bottles of laundry detergent. To gauge how much weight to lift when strength-training and toning: if you can perform 20 repetitions easily without getting tired, switch to heavier weights. If you can't do more than 5 or 6, switch to lighter weights.

Exercise or stability balls – these look like big beach balls. They are very inexpensive and are ideal for taking the stress from your back as you use them. They also put pressure on muscles from different angles so are more effective.

WHICH AEROBIC EXERCISE DOES WHAT

Walking – an excellent aerobic exercise especially if you haven't been very active and are building up your fitness levels. Pace needs to be brisk, but not so brisk that you cannot talk, and needs to be maintained for at least 30 minutes to start making a real difference.

Tips:
Try to incorporate some hills into the walk.
*Walking on grass will help absorb some of the
impact from your joints.*
Wear good walking boots or trainers.
Walk tall! Keep your back as straight as possible.
*As walking gets easier, break into a gentle jog for a
few minutes.*

Cycling – this is great for the body from the waist down, is gentle on the joints and an ideal aerobic workout that makes the heart pound, though it does show 5 to 10 heart beats lower than other aerobic exercises, so you will need to push yourself a little more to get into the Fat-Burning Zone. Cycling works best if

The Experts

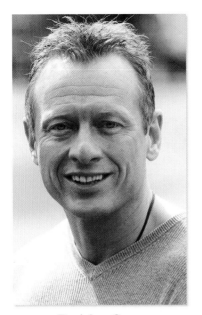

Dr Adam Carey

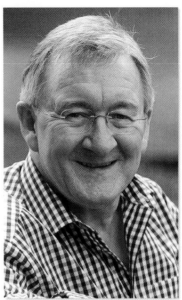

Dr Chris Steele

Harvey Walden

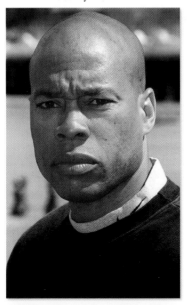

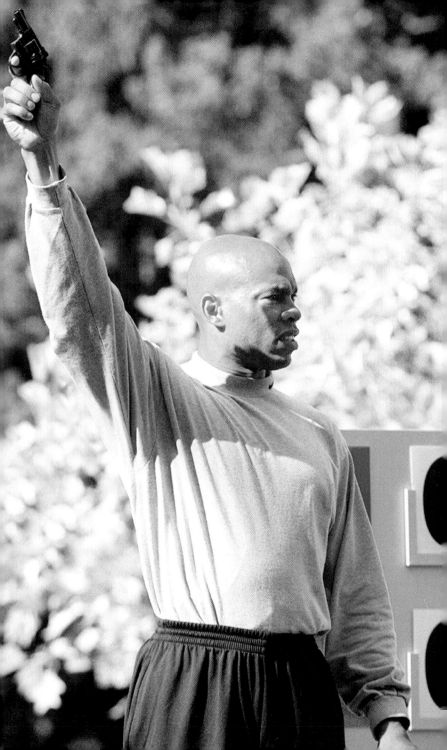

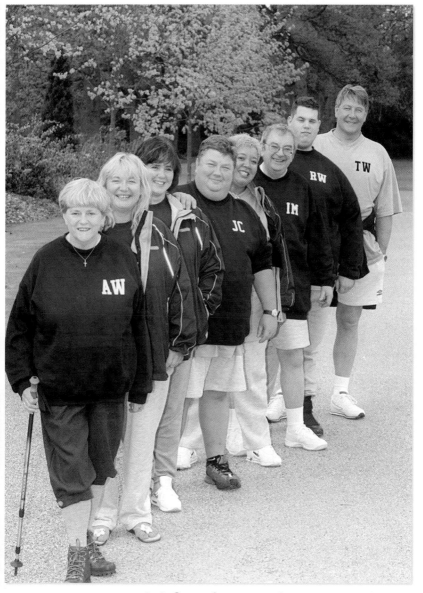

Left: Get ready, get set, go!

Above: The celebrities line up for the off. From the front: Ann
Widdecombe, Nicola Duffett, Coleen Nolan,
Jono Coleman, Kay Purcell, Ian McCaskill, Rik Waller, Tommy Walsh

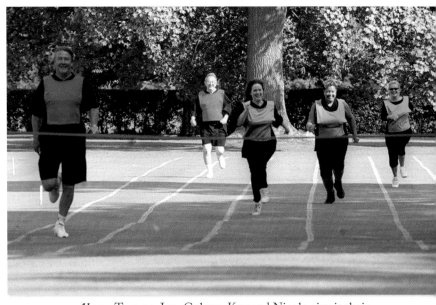

Above: Tommy, Ian, Coleen, Kay and Nicola give it their all in the running race

Below: Bend and stretch!

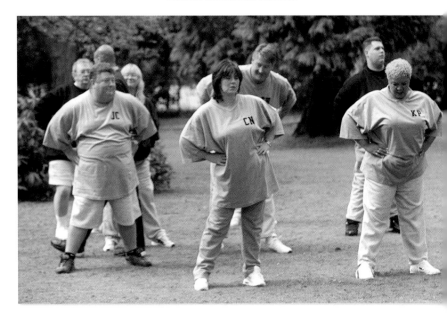

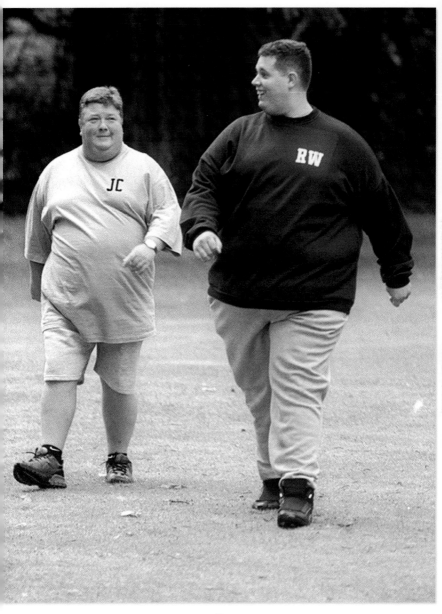

Above:
Jono and Rik stride out purposefully

Right: Ann and Rik reach out in Champneys grounds

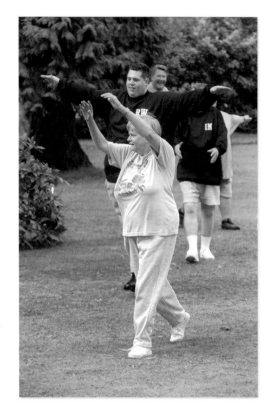

Below: Five go cycling: Ian, Kay, Nicola, Coleen and Tommy saddle up

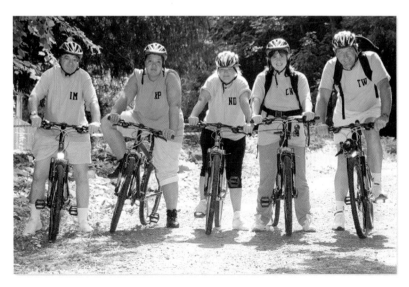

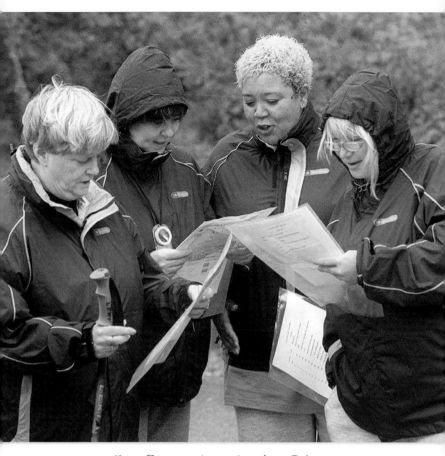

Above: Four go orienteering: Ann, Coleen, Kay and Nicola get co-ordinated

The Weigh-In 28 July 2002

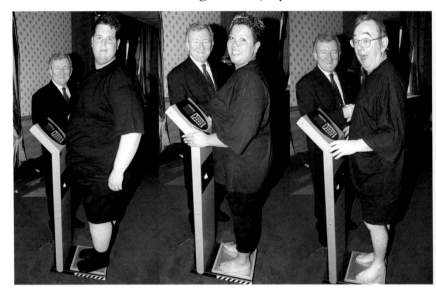

The moment of truth for
Rik, Kay, Ian, Nicola, Tommy and Coleen

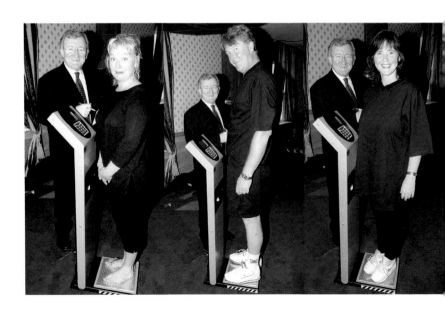

you combine it with other aerobic exercises and some upper body exercise on other days.

Tips:

Make sure you wear a helmet and visible clothing.

Comfortable cycling shorts will stop you getting saddle-sore.

Try to work out a route that includes some gentle hills.

If there are no hills, sprint for short periods, rising out of the saddle, to increase your exercise intensity.

Sit as straight in the saddle as possible, trying not to slouch.

Exercise bikes – these are ideal if road cycling is not an option (you can use a bike stand too – see above). It's worth investing in a good bike, though all can be set to differ the levels of intensity. Ian McCaskill loved his exercise bike: 'It helps me build up stamina and I can watch TV or listen to music which occupies the mind to pass the time.' Spinning Bikes (and there are normally classes at your health club) work on the whole body with varying resistance levels which increase and decrease the intensity levels by simulating hills.

Tips:

Proper cycling shorts are recommended and gel seat covers will make saddles even more comfortable.

Cycle to music or a TV programme and don't stop for commercial breaks!

Buy the best bike you can afford.

Jogging – the perfect exercise and the most effective and fastest way to burn fat. Jogging works the heart and the muscles and involves no equipment apart from a good pair of trainers. It can be hard on the joints though, especially when you begin jogging. Warm up first by running gently on the spot for five minutes and gently stretching the leg muscles, then run from heel to mid-foot to toe – Harvey suggests you visualize yourself 'running like a deer'. To build up your stamina, walk for five minutes, run for five, walk for five, run for five, until you find that it starts to become easier and you can run for longer. Build up to thirty minutes. It's very important to cool down afterwards by stretching the muscles again. Stretches should not be painful – if they are, you are not stretching properly.

Tips:

Harvey recommends you rotate your trainers and change them every six months or 500 miles, whichever is soonest, and that you wear cotton socks which will absorb sweat.

Make sure you drink plenty of water once you have finished running, and once you are running for a longer period, try to drink during the jog.

Don't be too ambitious. Build up your stamina slowly.

When sprinting, run more on your toes than on your heels.

Running on grass is easier on the joints than jogging on pavements.

Swimming – a non-weight bearing exercise which works all the muscle groups against the resistance of the water. It's a cheap way to exercise too if you use a public pool. However, swimming is not much of an aerobic, or fat-burning, exercise because you cannot swim at a high enough intensity to get into the *Fat-Burning Zone*. If you want to use swimming as your primary way of losing weight, combine it with a water aerobics class to get you into the *Fat-Burning Zone*, especially if you have joint problems.

Tips:

Warm up gently in the water before you start to swim more seriously, with two or three lengths at a gentle pace.

Vary your pace. Do one length fast, one length more slowly, and alternate the type of stroke.

Water aerobics classes are effective for muscle-strengthening and will stop you getting bored.

Rowing – a look at Sir Steve Redgrave will tell you just how good rowing is for the physique! It's an ideal cardiovascular (higher-intensity) workout, working all the major muscle groups, and has lower impact on the joints, as you are sitting down. The downside is that you need a river and a boat, or a rowing machine, and beginners can find it hard on the lower back.

Tips:

Breathe out as you pull back and breathe in as you move forward.

Wear shorts or cycling shorts to avoid getting clothes caught in the mechanism.

Alternate between working intensely then easing off.

Be careful of your lower back. Try not to lean too far as you pull back. Keep your back straight through out and use your legs, not your back.

Elliptical machines – these are a mixture of a tread-mill and a rowing machine, with poles that look like ski poles which you work as you walk. They are great for building stamina and working the whole body.

Tips:

As with rowing, alternate the intensity at which you work so that you don't tire yourself out.

Keep your arms relaxed, so that they do not tire before your legs do. Let your legs do most of the work.

Trampolining – Harvey calls this 'awesome!' Trampolines are easy on the joints and really get the heart racing, plus they are fun to exercise on. Small, low ones are not expensive and are an ideal way of exercising at home. You can jump as you watch TV or listen to some dance music.

Tips:

Use a mini trampoline – it's not so far to fall!

Trampoline to music, setting yourself a certain number of tracks before you stop.

Put it in front of the TV and work out for the length of a half-hour show.

Dancing – a great way to exercise which you can do at home to your favourite music. In fact, you only need to dance for six tracks on a CD and you've exercised for nearly half an hour! Choose vigorous and stirring music.

Tips:

Drink plenty of water after your dance session to make sure you do not dehydrate. Avoid alcohol if you are dancing at a club or party.

Stair-walking – another excellent exercise that you can do at home, either going up and down to music, or using the bottom few steps to go up and down, perhaps using handweights at the same time to work the upper body. Do it to music to keep you motivated.

Tips:

Be careful that you do not risk losing your step as you tire. Do the whole stairway to start with then work on the first one or two steps using them as you would a gym step.

Work your upper body using small dumb-bells or a couple of cans of beans (see exercises below).

Skipping – a popular exercise with boxers because it is great for agility. You may not have picked up a rope since school days, but it's easy to re-learn the skill. Skipping is a great aerobic work-out and fun to do.

Tips:

Start off slowly if you haven't skipped for a while, until you have re-learnt the technique.

Alternate between rates of intensity, working harder for 5 minutes, then slowing down for 5.

Skip to music with a strong rhythm.

HARVEY'S SUGGESTED WORKOUT

To exercise most effectively you will need to combine strength-building exercises with aerobic ones. This way you will burn fat and strengthen and tone up muscles too. There are lots of types of activity to choose from (see above). It's a question of picking what suits you and appeals to you, and varying activities so that you don't get bored. The only imperative is to warm up properly so that your muscles are ready to go and you are less likely to injure yourself, and to cool down properly afterwards.

NOTE: It's a good idea to do a low-intensity aerobic workout in one session, then a strengthening workout in another, but if you are going to do both on the same day, do the strengthening/toning one first. You will have upped your heart rate, so when you move on to aerobic exercise you will be burning fat almost straightaway. Having said that, it is better to do higher-intensity cardiovascular exercise before the strengthening exercises than to skip it altogether.

WARMING UP

This is an essential part of exercising because it not only gets your heart going, it also warms up the muscles and tendons, making them work more effectively and more flexibly. Start whatever exercise you choose to do slowly and gently – walking at a leisurely pace, jogging lightly – even on the spot – for about 5 to 10 minutes. You can even alternate jogging and walking. You should be sweating slightly but not out of breath.

Then gently stretch the muscles, concentrating on the ones you are going to use. Stretching increases your flexibility, which helps your overall fitness. Being flexible reduces the risk of injuring yourself, reduces muscle tension and soreness, helps you relax and increases the range in which you can move. Don't bounce or jerk when stretching – aim for a gradual, easy stretch. If you are running or cycling, work on the calves, hamstrings, quads, Achilles' tendon and the illiotibial (ITB) muscles (which go down over the hips to the side of the knees). Stretch for 15 to 30 seconds into the furthest position you can get into while still feeling comfortable.

THIGH STRETCH

This works on the adductor muscles which run down the inside of the thigh.

1. Stand sideways to a wall with your legs wide apart, wider than your shoulders, and with your feet facing forwards.

2. Bend your right knee, resting your hands on your bent knee and keeping your back straight. Hold for 10 seconds, return to standing position, then repeat bending your left knee.

You can vary this stretch by turning your feet out slightly and lunging gently in a rocking motion as you bend each knee.

HAMSTRING STRETCH

An important stretch to do before you start jogging or brisk walking, cycling or rowing.

1. Lie on your back, with your knees bent and your feet flat on the floor. Keeping your hips on the floor, lift up one leg with the flat of the foot towards the ceiling and hold your leg around the calf. Hold for 10 seconds then let your leg gently down to the floor.

2. Repeat with the other leg.

TRICEPS STRETCH

An easy stretch that you can even do sitting at your desk.

1. If standing, put your feet together and don't 'lock' your knees. Take one arm over your head and bend it down between your shoulder blades. With your other hand gently push the bent arm at the elbow until you can feel your triceps stretching. Hold for 10 seconds.

2. Repeat with the other arm.

SIDE STRETCH

This stretch works on all the muscles up the side of your body and arms, as well as the inter-costal muscles between the ribs.

1. Stand with your left hand resting at arm's length against a wall, at about shoulder height. Cross your left foot over your right.

2. Taking your weight on your right foot, push your hips away from the wall.

3. Bring your right arm over your head, touching the wall with this hand if you can, and hold for 10 seconds. Keep the weight on your right leg. You should be able to feel the stretch along the right side of your body from the thigh right up your arm. Repeat on the other side.

You can also do this stretch without a wall: simply stand with your feet wide apart, with one hand resting on your hip. Keeping your weight distributed evenly between both feet, bring your other arm over your head leaning gently to the side as you stretch.

FRONT THIGH STRETCH

The muscle at the front of your thigh – quadriceps – stretches every time you lift your leg. All athletes stretch this muscle before performing, and you can exercise it simply by kicking a football.

1. Holding on to the back of a sturdy chair with your right hand, stand with your feet together. Bend your left leg behind you until you can hold onto your foot with your left hand. Keep your legs together.

2. Now, keeping your left leg in that position, bend your right knee and tilt your body forwards. Your left knee will swing out backwards.

3. Straighten your right knee again and bring your body upright. Your left leg will still be swung out behind you and you should feel the stretch along the front of your thigh. Hold for 10 seconds then repeat with the other leg.

CAT STRETCH

This is a great stretch for the spine muscles around the vertebrae, which need to be kept supple to help ease and avoid back problems. If you have had back problems or injuries, do this exercise very carefully.

1. Go down on all fours with your arms the same distance apart as your shoulders, and your knees the same distance apart as your hips, keeping a straight vertical line between your bottom and your knees. Look straight ahead and arch your back downwards as far as is comfortable.

2. Drop your head down and at the same time arch your back upwards as fully as possible until you look like a cat stretching. Alternate this movement about 6 times.

CALF STRETCHES

There are powerful muscles in the calves which are put under pressure when you walk or run. If they are too tight they can hurt and cause problems with the Achilles' tendon at the back of the ankle.

1. Stand close to a wall, preferably next to a door jamb, so that you have something to hold on to. Put the ball of your foot against the wall, with the heel on the floor, and your other foot flat on the floor behind you. Push forward with your hips, lifting the heel of your back foot off the floor and keeping your front knee straight. Hold for 10 seconds and repeat with the other leg.

2. To stretch the lower calf muscles, stand at arm's length from the wall, resting the ball of your foot against the wall as before. Keeping your back foot flat on the floor and your back straight, bend the knee of your front leg, pushing it towards the wall. Hold for 10 seconds then repeat with the other leg.

INNER THIGH STRETCH

1. Sit on the floor holding the soles of your feet together and draw your feet in as far as is comfortable towards your crotch.

2. Keeping your back straight and holding your feet, gently push your knees down with your elbows towards the floor and hold for 10 seconds.

Aerobic Exercise

Pick from the aerobic exercises suggested on pages 128-133. You should try to exercise for at least 30 minutes to be effective, but build up your stamina slowly. Being too enthusiastic to begin with may result in injury and tire you out too quickly. Not only is this not an effective way of burning fat, it could also put you off the whole idea of exercising.

Vary the exercises you choose to do to stop yourself getting bored. This will also help you find an activity you really enjoy doing.

Cooling Down

Winding down is as important as warming up. Gradually downshift the intensity of your aerobic exercise: from a run, slow to a walk; from a brisk walk, slow to a slower pace, and so on. Once again do some stretching, working each muscle for about 30 seconds.

Strengthening/Toning:

These light weight-training exercises do not burn fat, but increase muscle mass which keeps up your metabolic rate. They work by including a high number of repetitions within each set. A set is a certain number of repetitions, followed by a short rest. Start at a rate of repetitions which is reasonably comfortable (you'll need to push yourself a bit), then increase the number as you get fitter and the exercises become easier – setting yourself personal targets will help – but aim to do the exercises *correctly* rather than trying to do a certain number each time. Remember to warm up the muscles before you start and breathe *out* with movements that involve exertion.

ADBOMINALS CRUNCHES

Toned abdominal muscles aren't just about a flat, six-pack stomach, they are an important support for the spine. Make sure you keep your hips and knees bent, so you are exercising the right muscles.

1. Lie flat on the floor on your back with either your knees bent and your feet flat on the ground or resting your lower legs on a sturdy chair (so your legs are at a 90° angle when bent). Place your hands lightly at the side of your head.

2. Contract your stomach muscles and raise your head and shoulders slightly off the ground, without pulling your head up with your hands.

3. Without touching the floor, crunch up and down, slowly moving your head towards your knees. Repeat in two sets of five, then return to your original position and rest.

Note: you may find it more comfortable to cross your arms across your chest or loosely cup your hands behind your neck.

Important: Do not anchor your feet under a chair, as this will exercise your thigh muscles not your abs.

CHAIR DIPS

One of Harvey's favourite exercises, which works on the back muscles as well as the triceps and pectorals on the arms and chest. Make sure the chair you use (a park bench will work too!) will not slip on the floor surface. Support yourself with both hands behind you on the chair with your arms straight but not locked. Stretch your legs out in front of you, resting on your heels.

By bending your elbows and keeping your body vertical, gently lower your body as far as feels comfortable, then push back up in one movement until your arms are straight again. Repeat 3 times, rest and then repeat 3 times again.

INNER THIGH

Great for strengthening and toning up the abductors, the muscles that bring the legs together.

1. Lie on your right side supporting your head in your right hand, and cross your left leg over your right knee so your foot is flat on the floor. Place your left hand in front of you to support yourself.

2. Lift your right leg as high as is comfortable and move it up and down without letting it touch the ground. Do not twist your body. Repeat 6 times, rest and repeat again 6 times.

3. Now do the same lying on your left side.

PRESS-UPS

These help develop firm arms and work the chest muscles. They are normally done keeping the legs and body in a straight line, but if you have not done them before (or for years) follow this routine:

1. Go down onto your hands and knees with your hands the same distance apart as your shoulders. Lift up your feet and cross your ankles.

2. Keeping your body straight, breathe out and bend your elbows, lowering your body towards the floor until your forehead is almost touching the ground, then lift again, breathing in. Repeat about 20 times or as often as you can comfortably.

CHEST-FIRMER

Do this using handweights/dumb-bells (see page 128 about choosing the right weights) or some cans of beans to the same weight. You can also support your upper body using an exercise ball.

1. Lie flat on the floor, or with your upper back, head and shoulders on the ball, and bend your legs with your feet flat on the floor. Hold a dumb-bell in each hand.

2. Start with hands upwards towards the ceiling, palms inwards. Open your arms until they are almost touching the floor either side of you, then bring them back up towards the ceiling again. Repeat 20 times or do as often as is comfortable.

BACK-TONER

This will shape and tone the muscles around the shoulder blades and upper back. Use handweights or improvize as before.

1. Stand with your feet shoulder-distance apart, without locking your knees and holding in your stomach. Hold a weight in each hand with your arms gently extended out to the sides, palms facing up and your elbows slightly behind your natural waistline.

2. Pull your elbows in towards each other behind your back as if you were trying to get your shoulder blades to meet. Relax your shoulders as you do this, but squeeze your shoulder blades. Hold for half a second then repeat. Aim to repeat this movement 12 times, in two sets.

KICKS

This is a great exercise for the bum and legs. Try to keep your upper body from swaying, and kick with control – don't throw your leg.

1. Stand with your feet together, then take a big step behind you with your right foot and bring it back to meet your left again.

2. As your feet meet, lift and kick forward with your left leg, lifting the knee and then extending the foot. Do this 12 times on each side.

Note: Keep your hands on your hips to help stabilize your upper body.

LOWER BACK

The lower back muscles need to be strong to avoid injury, and you need to build them up to balance out abdominal exercises. This exercise is just as effective if you use an exercise ball.

1. Lie on the floor on your front, and put your hands on your buttocks or by your side.

2. Keeping your chin in towards your chest, and your feet on the floor, lift up your torso, hold for a few seconds then lower again. Repeat as many times as is comfortable.

Note: While you're there, you can work on your buttocks! Rest your head on your hands and without raising your hips off the floor, lift your leg, keeping the toes pointed. Repeat 10 times, then repeat with the other leg.

ARM CURL

This exercise will develop and tone the biceps – you don't need to look like a body builder, but it is important to keep these muscles in shape. Use handweights or even a couple of bottles of laundry detergent, books or full carrier bags (weighing about 2-3kg).

1. Stand with your feet shoulder-distance apart, holding a weight in each hand, palms upward. Extend your arms towards the floor without locking your elbows.

2. Keep your wrists straight and lift your arms up to your shoulders, keeping your elbows into your waist. Hold for half a second and slowly lower again.

Note: An elastic exercise band is ideal for this: place your right foot in front on you and fix the elastic band beneath it. Holding the elastic in your hand, with the tension so that the arm curl is just possible, bend your elbow up towards your chest. (Keep your back straight and remember to keep your elbows tucked in.) Hold for a few seconds and lower. Repeat 10 times, in three sets. Repeat using the other arm and leg.

On page 214 you'll find a helpful chart for you to record your exercise routine and rates. Use it to amaze yourself at your growing strength and stamina.

CHAPTER 6

YOUR QUESTIONS
ANSWERED

The beauty of *Fit Club* lay in its simplicity. No complicated calorie-counting or food juggling. No elaborate and contorting exercises to tackle. We hope the programme is clear and easy to follow, but just in case, we've asked the experts to answer some of the most common concerns that crop up during a weightloss regime.

About exercise
What if I cycle to the shops for 15 minutes then get back on the bike to come home? Will I still benefit from aerobic exercise?
Harvey says: It really won't benefit you in terms of burning fat by getting off after 15 minutes then getting back on again. You are working on a different type of exercise or conditioning by doing that – more like anaerobic exercise. It's like doing 15 sprints and calling it a day. You are working on speed and explosiveness rather than on exercise at a sustainable fat-burning level. That's why it's so important to pace yourself when you are trying to burn fat and that is the main reason why heart monitors are ideal to use when exercising. These help you to see the level at which your heart is working, and, once you know your maximum heart rate (see pages 123-124), it will tell you whether you are exercising at the right intensity for burning fat.

However, a trip to the shops on a bike, however long it takes, is vastly better for you than going in the car!

Can I just diet or just do exercise?

Chris says: Many people wonder why they are over-weight when they claim to hardly eat a thing. It's because they hardly do a thing! Dieting will help you lose pounds, but eating normally and taking some form of exercise is the healthiest, most effective way to sustained weightloss. By doing something as simple as walking for 30 minutes every day, whatever the weather, you will be exercising your heart, strengthening your muscles and helping to shift excess pounds. Do this whilst following a lower fat diet, with plenty of healthier food options, and you are on the road to success!

I have a bad back and bad joints. Which exercises will help and which should I avoid?

Harvey says: If you have a bad back, but have been cleared by a GP to engage in exercise, then activity that involves you using your lower back – such as rowing, squats, press-ups – should be avoided or done with caution and light weights. It really depends on how bad the injury is and what you know you can tolerate, as well as what your GP has said you can do. Even lunges and running can be hard on someone with a bad back. Good options would be exercises like swimming, riding a stationary bike or even using an elliptical machine. Walking, too, is a good idea.

As far as bad joints are concerned, choose low-impact exercises like cycling, swimming, walking on a treadmill, yoga, tai chi, using an elliptical machine. Again, weigh up the severity of the injuries and talk to your GP. My best story about knowing when your body is telling you, 'Hello, dummy, I am hurt, give yourself a break' happened in 1999. I was playing football and training for the marathon. I took a pretty bad hit on my shin but thought it was a bruise and continued to run 50 miles a week through the pain. After finally going to the doctor and having an X-ray, it turned out I had a stress fracture and I wound up on crutches!

I am very busy and can't find the time to go to the gym. Is there a good weightloss exercise that I can do at home?

It's great to be keen to exercise despite a busy schedule, and if you look at your day, you may find you do have half an hour here or there for a run. However, there is plenty of good aerobic (weightloss) exercise you can do at home – one of the best is skipping. Try not to do it on hard surfaces – grass or a wooden floor would be better – and don't jump too high, just high enough for the rope to pass under your feet. Contact the British Rope Skipping Association (www.brsa.org.uk) on 01527 854194.

I have just spent a lot of money on a pair of trainers, yet I am still getting blisters. Why?

The problem may be your socks. As your feet sweat they cause friction. Invest in a pair of sports socks which are 100 per cent cotton, and preferably a pair which have two thin layers so they rub against each other, not your skin.

I go to a gym, but am about to go on holiday where there is a pool. I want to keep exercising. How can I make sure I get the best from swimming?

Alternate your swimming between lengths, varying your speed and stroke each time, and tone up with some exercises using the water resistance. Move your arms and legs in an arc shape 'pushing' the water away as you move. Another routine is to hold on to the edge of the pool, with your back against the side, and lift your legs up to your stomach keeping your hips against the wall. Do this 5 times, for 3 sets.

I am 55 and want to start exercising, but don't fancy a gym and certainly not an aerobics class. What can I do?

Brisk walking is an excellent exercise especially for those who are a little out of practice. It burns over 300 calories an hour and requires only a good pair of walking shoes. Walking works the heart and lungs and tones up the body below the waist. The British Heart Foundation have an initiative called 'Walking the Way to Health'. Go to www.whi.org.uk or call 01580 200443.

Is it possible to get a flatter stomach just through toning exercise?

Certainly exercises which concentrate on the abdominal muscles will help tone the stomach (see pages 139-140), but a big stomach is also due to fat. Aerobic exercise combined with a healthy low-fat diet will help to burn the fat from this area.

Should I be tucking my feet under something when I do crunching exercises on my stomach?
This method of anchoring the feet can put strain on your lower back and work the thigh muscles rather than the abdominal ones that you are aiming at. Follow the routine on pages 139-140, which suggests resting your lower legs on the seat of a chair or leaving your feet (and your hips) on the floor.

I have been exercising and eating healthily but have put on a pound in a week. Help!
This can seem demotivating, but it is actually a direct result of strengthening and building up muscles which weigh more than fat. Make sure you are doing plenty of fat-burning (aerobic) as well as muscle-strengthening exercises, and maintain a healthy, low-fat diet and you will find that your weight will continue on a downward trend.

I have been told by friends that the best way to work out is with aerobic activity and weight training, and to push myself hard. Is this right?
This mix of exercise is ideal, as you will have found out by reading Chapter 5. However, you should never push yourself until you are too tired to go on. Not only will this put you at greater risk of injury, it is very likely to put you off exercise all together! Do just enough so that you feel you could always do a bit more. You should never be so out of breath that you feel ill or find it hard to talk. Start off at a gentle pace, and build up until it feels comfortable, but your heart and muscles are working well.

Diet and food

Is the Fit Club way of eating suitable for overweight children?

It's a very suitable way of helping overweight children obtain the nutrients they need for growth and repair, while providing them with plenty of energy. It will also help to control carbohydrate cravings that so often lead them to binge on easily available snack foods, like crisps, sweets and biscuits. In fact, it provides an ideal healthy way of eating for anyone for life, so introducing this healthy balanced diet in childhood is one of the best favours you could ever do for your kids.

When adapting the advice in this book for children, however, use Adam's 80/20 plan, in which 80 per cent of meals are based around the eating scheme and 20 per cent are more relaxed, allowing for trips to restaurants with friends and other less balanced meals, rather than the stricter 95/5 plan recommended for adults during their initial weightloss phase. And because children burn up so much energy, by just growing and being active, around 70 per cent of their calorie intake should be from carbohydrates, as opposed to the 55 per cent recommended for adults.

Learning to eat healthily is of vital importance to young people, and habits formed early will last a lifetime – for better or worse. Just make sure children eat a wide variety of good quality foods from all the food groups, and they'll soon come to see junk food for what it really is – just junk! Try to involve them in the preparation of food, too. They will often be more willing to eat something new if they have had a hand in making it!

Very obese children should always have specialized help, so if your child is very overweight don't try to rectify things yourself. Contact your doctor for advice.

Most diets count calories. Why not this eating programme?

Adam feels strongly that this way of eating should be easy to incorporate into your daily life, so he gave the celebrities a quick and easy way of calculating how much food is right for them. It doesn't involve any specialized equipment, and you can do it anywhere. All you need is your hands! It involves judging quantities of food in relation to the size of the palm of one hand, minus fingers and thumb, and it is fully explained in Chapter 4.

I cannot eat nuts. Is there a good alternative which provides the same level of nutrition?

There are many other excellent sources of high-grade protein. Fish, lean meat and poultry, eggs, seeds, soya products and cheese can all be used to ring the changes in your protein intake.

I am vegetarian. How can I ensure I am getting enough protein without resorting to fatty foods?

You are right to be careful about the type of protein you eat. Many vegetarians rely on cheese to supply the protein they need, but dairy produce can be high in saturated fats. Try alternatives such as eggs, tofu and other soya products, nuts and seeds and fish, if you eat it. Varying your sources of nutrition as much as possible gives you the best chance of having a truly healthy, balanced diet.

Help! I couldn't resist temptation and just wolfed down a huge junk food meal. What can I do?

Don't panic. As Adam says, you are only ever one meal away from eating healthily, so although you gave in, don't give up. You can regard this as one of the meals where you allow yourself to relax, the 5 part of the 95/5 plan or part of the 20 in 80/20. A single slip-up wasn't responsible for your being overweight in the first place – it's what you eat the rest of the time that counts. In practical terms, you might find the scales show an increase, but this will be mostly due to water retention. Return to your normal balanced, healthy eating, drink plenty of water and you'll be back on track in no time.

More importantly, however, you can use this experience as a learning tool. Why do you think it happened? Did you allow yourself to become too hungry by skipping snacks or eating insufficient protein at each meal? Were you stressed or bored? Had you missed an exercise session? If you can pin down the reason, you can help yourself to avoid similar problems in the future. How did the meal make you feel once you'd eaten it? Not as good as you were expecting it to, in all probability. Once you've started to give your body the balanced nutrition it needs, you'll find your appetite is not satisfied by junk food. That's progress!

CHAPTER 7

WHEN IT GOES
ALL PEAR-SHAPED!

Taking the decision to start a weightloss programme is a great and courageous step forward. Actually starting it is even better. In those first days, your resolve is strong. You feel good that you've finally done something about a problem that has almost certainly been troubling you for years. Your intentions are clear, your mind is made up and you're full of enthusiasm. Terrific! Enjoy this stage in your new healthier lifestyle. But remember that it is only the start. There will be times when the way ahead does not look so clear, obstacles may obstruct your way and your motivation may falter. And that is what this chapter is all about.

With the *Fit Club* plan, some of the changes you are making will form the basis of the new, healthier habits that should last you a lifetime – which is why it makes so much more sense than previous fad diets you may have tried – and although these changes will have undeniably positive results, they may still be hard to stick with. You are bound to encounter many points in your journey towards a healthy weight and regular exercise regime when your old habits resurface, or when circumstances conspire to make it hard for you to eat and to work out as you know you should.

But setbacks are normal. It's how you react to them that makes the crucial difference between success and failure. Plan for obstacles. Accept them. Be prepared to cope with them. Facing your setbacks and problems and overcoming them, rather than giving up at the first sign of a problem, will become a habit, and one you should be proud to cultivate.

Obstacles will arise from many, sometimes unexpected sources. Circumstances can change: work schedules, holidays, injuries, parties – all these can cause havoc in an otherwise well organized regime. Other people can cause problems, sometimes even deliberately sabotaging your best efforts, sometimes unwittingly by expecting you to act as you would have done in the past. Sometimes, let's face it, you'll just get fed up and mutiny against your own carefully laid plans.

We've tried to highlight the danger points that occur in most people's lives. These are the moments when you need some extra help. Times when, perhaps in the past, you would have chucked the whole thing in. Not this time. Remember, you're not alone. Everyone who has ever undertaken the kind of life-change you and all the members of *Fit Club* have committed to will have had times when their resolve slipped. The extra strategies, tactics, affirmations and approaches we've collected in this chapter will help you find your way.

Dispelling the dieting myths

Most people who are trying to lose weight will tell you that they've tried every diet imaginable to shed the pounds. As *Fit Club* has proved, many of these are faddy diets which left us exactly where we started – overweight. This is because trendy diets are often devised to provide a quick fix, not slower, sustainable weightloss, so we are fed half-truths and bogus science.

Here are a few popular myths:

Diet myth no. 1 – All dietary fat is bad

If you are trying to lose weight, it is a good idea to reduce the fat in your diet because fat provides more calories than either carbohydrate or protein (gram for gram fat provides 9, protein 4 and carbohydrate 3.75). In fact, even if you don't need to lose weight, reducing your fat intake to less than 35 per cent of your total calorie intake is recommended for good health. Adam's plan reduces fat intake to about 15 per cent, but the choice of fats is critical. Saturated fats (animal fats) in the diet can increase blood cholesterol levels, increasing risk of heart disease, whereas monounsaturates, polyunsaturates and fats from oily fish can help reduce risk of heart disease. Some fat in your diet is important so don't cut it out completely and include some each day.

Diet myth no. 2 – Fat can be lost rapidly

Very often when people start to diet they find that they can lose vast amounts of weight in the first week and then the weightloss slows down. This is when they start to feel demoralized and often give up, only to repeat the cycle a few weeks later when the next 'must-have' diet hits the magazines. Fat we store in our bodies cannot be lost rapidly, but increasing your protein intake and reducing refined carbs makes it easier for your body to use up the fat you have stored.

Diet myth no. 3 – You can spot-reduce fat, particularly on the hips and thighs

As unfair as it may seem, there is not much we can do

about the sites from which we gain and lose weight. Some diets advocate extremely low-fat, low-calorie diets to target these so called 'problem' areas. Very low-calorie diets have been criticized by the Department of Health as being potentially dangerous. It is recommended that a person should not go below 800 calories per day. It is much better to eat a healthy, balanced diet that you enjoy and take up some form of enjoyable exercise that you can do regularly. With muscle-toning exercises, you can then target areas which need particular attention, like the tummy or thighs. See Chapter 5.

Diet myth no. 4 – You shouldn't mix protein foods and carbohydrate foods at the same meal

Dr. William Hay came up with the theory of 'food combining' at the beginning of the last century. He believed that disease resulted from the accumulation of toxins and acid waste in our bodies. The way to cure disease, he reckoned, was to avoid eating 'foods that fight'. By this he meant that you should not mix proteins and carbohydrates in the same meal, and that you should eat foods which restore the body's natural balance between acids and alkalis. However, there is no scientific evidence whatsoever to support this theory and we know now that you should eat some protein at every meal to provide long-lasting energy. This kind of diet may appear to work because intake is restricted, but it is not sustainable or balanced.

Diet myth no. 5 – Your blood group dictates which foods you should and shouldn't eat

Diets based on the idea that your blood group can dictate which foods are likely to cause weight gain have no scientific basis. The idea behind these diets is to split foods into groups which are 'highly beneficial', 'neutral' and 'to be avoided'. You may well lose weight on this diet because it is so restrictive, but in being so it is also likely to be unbalanced. Daily consumption of fruit and vegetables of all types should be encouraged to help prevent diseases such as heart disease and cancer.

Diet myth no. 6 – Healthy eating costs more

One of Adam Carey's major points is that we don't take enough time to ensure that our diet is healthy and balanced. His argument is that relying on prepared foods that are often high in fat, salt and additives is actually a far less healthy and certainly more expensive option than cooking meals ourselves. Take a look at Adam's list of suggested meals and snacks in Chapter 5, and the recipes in Chapter 9 and you'll see that they offer tasty and far healthier options than ready meals and prepared snacks. Certainly, cooking is more effort initially than microwaving ready meals but it should be far less expensive, and once you organize yourself to cook larger quantities and freeze ahead you may even find your food bill goes down, not up. Compare the prices: supermarket cook-chilled meals cost about £3-4. For that price you could buy two chicken breasts, a bag of salad and some new potatoes.

Preparing to face problems

Recognize any of these problems along the way? Here's how to tackle them and get yourself through.

I'm feeling deprived!

Don't regard this as a time of deprivation. You are doing something very positive for your body, probably treating it well for the first time in years. Treat your body as though your life depended on it – because, guess what, it does!

Treat your body better, not just in how you eat and exercise, but with small gestures that make you feel and look better. Aim for three acts of kindness to your body each day. It could be as simple as taking a vitamin supplement, body brushing before your shower, taking time to relax and stretch before bed. Make these into a habit, and after a month you'll have given your body almost 100 little treats. And it will show!

Start visualizing yourself as a slim, strong and healthy person, instead of focusing on the parts of your body that you think look too fat. Remember to keep looking at that old photograph of how you used to look when you were slimmer (as suggested in Chapter 3). Think of yourself moving towards being that way again.

I can't resist temptation

When you feel tempted to overeat or to skip your exercise, don't panic or block out the feeling. You'll still feel compelled to overeat in circumstances when you've done so in the past, whether it's at dinner parties or Sunday lunches, but working through this, using some of the suggestions below, will help you create a new association in your mind between food and good habits. You're bound to feel like missing out on your workout sometimes. Everybody does. And it's all too easy to create excuses, but the feel-good effect you experience when you overcome your reluctance and push forward consistently with your exercise plan will reinforce your confidence in your ability to break through the barriers you've erected in the past.

Help! I'm standing in front of the fridge but I've just had a meal

If you find yourself reaching for a snack when you know you're not even hungry, you're in danger of slipping back into your old habits and undoing all your good work. Before you dip anything in mayonnaise, try one of our tried and tested strategies for avoiding this kind of pointless snacking.

• Try to analyse how you feel. Are you bored, depressed, anxious, tired, trying to avoid getting on with something else? Or do you just want something to chew? If you can find another way of coping with the way you feel, you'll have made important progress in changing your eating habits for the better.

• Try to break that habit by exercising instead. It does not have to be intense exercise. Sometimes a quiet stroll can have a great impact on relieving stress. Or divert yourself by doing some physical activity around the house or garden.

• Drink a glass of water first. Sometimes you may be thirsty rather than hungry but you've forgotten how to recognize the signals.

• Put on a favourite song and listen to it while relaxing. It can lift your mood and divert you enough to let the food craving pass.

• Resolve to go away for 10 minutes to wait and see if you really do want something to eat. If at the end of that time you still want it as much, then choose a healthy, tasty snack (see below).

• Clean your teeth!

• Have a stick of sugar-free gum.

• If you just have to have something to chew on or to taste, choose something like celery or raw carrot, or something with a clear, strong flavour that lasts in your mouth, like a cube of strong cheese or a couple of olives.

• Tackle whatever it is you know you're trying to avoid – whether it's filling in a tax return, making a difficult phone call, or doing the ironing. You know you'll feel better once it's done.

• Try a few of Harvey's toning exercises – give it 110 per cent!

• Sit down and do some deep-breathing exercises. This is particularly useful if you think the reason you want to eat is because you are stressed or tired.

• Keep a note of the times you feel like eating for reasons other than hunger, and of the solutions you find for diverting yourself. It can help you build up an awareness of how you really feel, plus a repertoire of diversions that work. If you find yourself craving a particular food at the same time every day, think about indulging yourself in a small way, once in a while. For example, a couple of squares of really good quality chocolate mid-afternoon can be the kind of treat that

will keep you on track with your healthy eating.
• Phone a friend, particularly one who will support you and help with your motivation, and have a good chat.
• Read a book or magazine.
• Try an exercise video, particularly one with a short routine you can fit in without disrupting your plans for the rest of the day.
• Take a shower, using some lovely products that will make you feel pampered and rewarded.
• If you really are tired – try a nap.

I get hungry between meals

Following Adam Carey's advice in Chapter 4 should ensure that you never feel so hungry that you overeat or binge on foods that you know are bad for you. Combining protein with complex carbohydrates will satisfy you for longer and allow you to regain control of the way you eat. Even sugar cravings start to subside after about 48 hours of eating according to the plan. Regulate your appetite using the between-meal snacks suggested in Chapter 4, and keep the blood-sugar roller coaster at bay.

I've just got to have...

Having moments when you've just got to give in to a craving for something a bit less healthy? As Adam Carey stressed in Chapter 4, there is no such thing as bad food, and nothing is forbidden on his eating plan. This is what makes it so much easier to stick with than the unrealistically strict crash diets we've all tried and failed at. You're less likely to have cravings because you're not denying yourself anything, so you should find your appetite more regular and easier to control. But for whatever reason, we all sometimes long for something naughty but nice.

By all means, give in to temptation now and again. Give in, but never give up. Thinking hard about how you feel when a craving overtakes you, and planning ahead so you can cope is the way to succeed.

If you are experiencing regular cravings, keep a diary to try to identify the trigger. Anxiety, tiredness and stress are all emotional triggers that can set off cravings, and once you have some insight into what sets you off, you can start addressing the cause rather than the symptom.

If you know when most of your cravings strike, make sure you have a small portion of what you fancy to hand during this time or, if you want to beat it, change your routine during the time you tend to get cravings.

If chocolate is your thing, plan for a treat by buying yourself one or two really good quality chocolates. You'll relish the flavour far more than if you scoffed down a whole bar of a cheaper brand.

For salt cravings, try a small cube of feta cheese, a few spiced almonds, a sliver of really good Parmesan or a handful of cherry tomatoes. Aim to give yourself a small but really delicious flavour hit that will satisfy you when you most need it.

If you want something really sweet, keep peeled bananas in the freezer and put them in a blender for a healthy version of ice cream. Mix in a tablespoon of yogurt or cottage cheese to add protein. You'll feel like you indulged, but you didn't.

I deserve and want a treat!

You certainly do, but you need to work beyond the mindset of rewarding yourself with food. This is short-term thinking and is the downfall of anyone who throws themselves into a crash diet. If you are sticking to your healthy eating and exercise plan you deserve better than to spoil it all with a splurge. The best way to cope with this kind of thinking is to set yourself a target – for example, going to the gym regularly for two weeks, losing 1 kg a week for a month, sticking with your eating plan for a week – and plan your reward in advance. Set both small-scale and larger targets and make the reward fit the accomplishment. It could be as small as a bag of cherries; for a bigger reward, buy yourself a new CD, tickets to a film or sporting fixture. When you've reached your goal, plan to treat yourself to a weekend away or to buy something you want for your house. The best reward of all, of course, is buying yourself clothes a size or two smaller than you're wearing at the moment.

I'm going to a party. How can I avoid a binge?

Whether you're throwing a party yourself or going to someone else's, you're moving into dangerous territory. However, you can still have fun while avoiding the temptation of rich dips and high-fat snacks.

• Plan ahead: If you're going to a party straight after work, eat something before you go so that you don't dive into the nearest plate of snacks when you arrive. Go for something filling, such as a sandwich, a bowl of wholegrain cereal or one of Adam Carey's delicious and satisfying snacks.

• Choose wisely: If you haven't got time to eat before the party, choose what you eat carefully. Breadsticks or pumpernickel are a great choice but watch out for those dips. An average portion of houmous contains 6g fat and 90 calories compared with the same amount of taramasalata that has 25g fat and 250 calories. Stick with celery, carrot sticks and cherry tomatoes and you can't go wrong.

• Drink a glass of water: If you haven't got time to eat and want to resist snacks completely, then drink a glass of water to help fill your stomach and keep your hunger at bay.

• Sugar-free gum: Chewing gum is a great, if not very elegant, way to stop you nibbling bits of food while you're cooking.

• Watch the alcohol: Although alcohol contains no fat, a small glass of wine can set you back 132 calories, and if you feel a little light-headed you can find your willpower sadly eroded. To keep the calorie-count down, try alternating wine with mineral water. Or try gin and tonic, but without the gin – lots of ice and lemon with refreshing tonic – and you probably won't even be able to tell the difference.

• Be ruthless: Don't leave bowls of unfinished snacks lying around. Throw them out (or get someone else to do it for you) as soon as your guests have left. Remember, even a few handfuls of crisps could hugely increase your intake of fat and refined carbs.

I'm losing interest in exercise. How can I get back on track?

Everybody gets fed up with their exercise regime after

a while. Be prepared for this happening and work through those feelings of apathy. When you see the results, you'll be encouraged to redouble your efforts. See Chapters 5 and 6 for ways to stay motivated.

• Keep focused on your goal. Imagine what it would be like to be fit and a healthy weight. Imagine how you will feel. Imagine what you will do with all the new energy you have. You have to keep focused on the positive. When you don't feel like going to the gym, just think of the results you will achieve if you make the effort.

• Keep track of your achievements. You are dieting and exercising for a reason. Concentrate on the pounds you've lost, the extra distance you can swim, or how you can now keep up with everyone else in that exhausting aerobics class.

• Make your weightloss real. Go to the supermarket and look at the equivalent weight you have lost in lard. Remember to try the backpack test (page 80) and fill it with the weight you have lost using tins of beans or bags of sugar. Try picking it up and carrying it around for a while for a scary reminder of what you used to have to carry around permanently.

• Break your goals down into manageable steps. For instance, don't just say, 'I want to lose 50 pounds and run a 10-minute mile'. Split these goals down into smaller pieces. For instance, in the next six months, you can plan to lose 10lbs and actually be able to jog a mile. When you make a number of smaller accomplishments, you feel good about yourself because you can think about what you *have* accomplished, not what you have *not* accomplished.

• Adopt the same attitude as with your eating plan –
you can give in, but don't give up. There's no limit to
the number of chances you will get to start exercising
again. If you miss a session or two, you can easily get
going again. The chances are, if you skip your exercise
session, you'll actually feel less energetic, and that will
help to remind you that one of the best incentives for
exercising is how great it makes you feel straightaway.
• Be sure to reward yourself when you have achieved a
goal. See above for inspiration on non-food rewards.

I just don't have time to exercise

This is the classic excuse for people who would really
prefer not to do anything. There is always time to
include some extra activity if you really want to, and
in Chapter 5 you'll have found plenty of ways to exercise at home. To keep your exercise regime going
through thick and thin, you may have to do some
careful planning, and sometimes you have to use the
ploys on pages 167-169 to get through those days
when your motivation flags and you'd really rather
take a break. The most important thing about your fitness programme is that you should enjoy it, or you'll
need willpower as strong as Harvey's to keep yourself
at it. Despite the fact that Harvey gets up every morning at 4am to run his daily eight miles, he hates running and finds it boring. 'I stick with it because it's the
most efficient way for me to work out before I even
start working,' he says. For mere mortals, however, it's
really safer to choose something you know you'll
enjoy. Remind yourself by re-reading Chapter 5.

I've joined a gym and find my motivation is flagging
It's a common occurrence and an expensive one. Here are a few ways to get you back on the straight and narrow.

• Designate an area of your car as your 'sports locker'. Keep a pair of tennis shoes there, or your roller blades and knee pads, a couple of pairs of clean socks, a clean towel, some wet wipes, a frisbee, tennis rackets, a football or a skipping rope, whatever takes your fancy. This way, whenever you have a little extra time you can be spontaneous. This is a fun way to break up the monotony and do something that's fun and unexpected, either on your own or with the whole family.

• Choose a gym that is between your home and your work, or the kids' school, or the shops so you don't have to go out of your way to get there. If you can drop in on your way to or from somewhere else you're far more likely to stick with it.

• Calculate how much your workout will cost you if you go once a week, twice a week, three times – and so on. Clearly, the more often you go, the better value you are getting for your subscription.

• If you've resolved to go, say, three times a week and it works out at 50p a visit, keep a piggy bank and drop in the same amount if you ever miss.

• Make sure your gym has convenient parking – you don't want to give yourself a ready-made excuse for not going.

• Remember Harvey's tip: splash out on some workout gear that makes you feel and look your best. Then think about how much better you'll be looking in a month or so.

• If your gym is running a sponsored workout or challenge, sign up for it. This worked for the celebrities at the *Fit Club*, who were prepared to make the effort for a charity when they may not have gone to the same lengths for themselves.

• Write your gym session into your diary, just as if it were an appointment or date and decide on regular times to go, if possible.

• Set an alarm clock to ring half an hour before you are due at the gym, to give you plenty of time to finish off whatever you're doing and get ready.

Ask a supportive friend or your partner to give you a call to remind you when you have to go to the gym. Having someone else involved makes it harder to bunk off.

• If you don't feel like a workout, make yourself go to the gym anyway just for a swim and a sauna. The chances are that once you've gone to the trouble of getting yourself there, you'll do more.

• Get to know the staff by name. It's a great morale-booster when they greet you every time you arrive.

• If your gym has lockers, make sure you leave something important there, like a work jacket or your deodorant, so you'll have a reason to go back.

• Treat yourself to some special shower gel and shampoo, so that you'll come to associate your workouts with the pleasure of using them.

• If you are going out in the evening, don't wash your hair first thing. Go to the gym at lunchtime and wash it there after your workout.

• Take advantage of the different classes on offer at the gym. If you can fit in an extra session of, say, spinning, Pilates or step every couple of weeks, it helps keep your interest going and offers a new challenge to keep you on your toes.

• Ask the instructor to vary your programme every six weeks or so. Your muscles accommodate a regular regime after a while and you no longer get the full benefit. Regular small changes help to keep your body in peak condition.

• Make a chart and put it somewhere very visible. Tick off the days you do go to the gym, but put a big cross by the days you don't go.

• Award yourself a treat every time you manage to go eight times in a row without missing a session. A massage, some new shorts or a pedometer will help spur you on to even greater efforts.

• Get someone to take a photo of you every couple of weeks, wearing your exercise gear, so you can see the difference your exercise programme is making.

• Arrange to meet a friend after your session somewhere near the gym.

I'm going on holiday – does it have to wreck my exercise regime?

It's very common to use going away as an excuse to give up on your fitness plan, but people who are naturally active and fit find many new ways to keep moving on holiday – so there really is no reason why anyone trying to become more active should give up. With a bit of forward planning, you can continue and even increase your healthy exercise programme, and since you don't have to work, and are on a completely different schedule, it's the ideal time to try something new. A change of scene, plenty of fresh air and some new activities could make all the difference to your appearance. By the time you go home, you should be looking better than ever!

• Probably the easiest way to continue your training is to use the on-site fitness facility in your hotel. Ask for details of what is available, and book some exercise classes and time in the gym. It's an ideal time to try something new like water aerobics, and to pamper yourself in a sauna or steam bath.

• Smaller hotels may not have fitness centres on-site, but they often have agreements with local health clubs to allow guest privileges. Even if your hotel has no arrangements with a local club, you may be able to use a facility for a nominal guest fee. Check the local phone book, or ask the hotel concierge to advise you.

• If you belong to a health club, ask before you leave for your trip if there is a branch where you are going, or an affiliate programme that will allow you to become a temporary member of a club at your destination.

• It may appeal more to you to exercise at your convenience in your hotel room. Wake up early and exercise with a video you have brought from home or have rented from the hotel, or use the exercises in Chapter 5, all of which are designed for use at home.

• Pack collapsible handweights and fill them with water for an in-room strength training workout. Check your local sports shop for collapsible dumb-bells, elastic bands and other exercise equipment made specifically for travel.

• On beach holidays, try running on dry sand or wading through thigh-deep water to add an extra challenge. Swim whenever you can.

• Use the resistance of water for your strengthening exercises. Warm up with a couple of lengths, then mimic the exercises in Chapter 5 in the water.

• Buy a Frisbee or a ball and play with it on the beach whenever it's not too crowded or hot.

• Book in for an hour of tennis at a local court, or hire bikes, take a skipping rope to the beach, walk everywhere and, provided the weather is not too hot, continue your running programme.

• Aim to maintain your current level at least, to keep your healthy lifestyle intact – there is no reason to slip back while you're on holiday. You could even extend what you normally do.

Holiday exercise safety tips

Regardless of where you will be exercising, always take the following safety precautions:

• Carry identification with your name and address, as well as the name and telephone number of the place where you will be staying.

• Dress for the climate and drink water to keep yourself properly hydrated. Monitor your heart rate and exertion level during exercise to be sure you aren't exceeding your physical limitations.

• As always, exercise safely and within your fitness level, remembering that travel can take its toll on the body as a result of stressors like changes in time zones, climate and daily schedules. While exercise may help some people cope with these changes, other people may need to slow down a bit.

CHAPTER 8

CHAMPNEYS RECIPES

At *Fit Club*, the celebrity members were encouraged by Adam Carey to enjoy their meals and to eat regularly. Nothing was banned, starvation was not an option, and the members, to their amazement, found that they could eat healthy, balanced and satisfying meals – and still lose weight!

While they were at Champneys, the celebrities relished the delicious menus created by resident chef, Adam Palmer. Now you can sample some of his specially devised recipes too. As tasty as they are satisfying, they offer the combination of nutrients that ensures healthy, sustainable weightloss. Perfect for entertaining, but with a few simple alterations to the ingredients, you can adapt them for everyday family meals.

Key to symbol for recipes:

♥   – very low fat (5 g or less per serving)
      – unsaturated fats

🍎   – low fibre (2 g or less per serving)
 🍎🍎   – medium fibre (2-5 g per serving)
🍎🍎🍎   – high fibre (over 5 g per serving)

BREAKFASTS

Banana, citrus and oat smoothie
Serves 4
50 g/2 oz **rolled oats**
100 ml/3½ fl oz **skimmed milk**
3 small **bananas**
finely grated zest and juice of 1 **orange**
finely grated zest and juice of 1 **lemon**
150 ml/5 fl oz **low-fat yogurt**
150 ml/5 fl oz **low-fat fromage frais**
3 tablespoons **clear honey**
pinch of **mixed spice**
8 **ice cubes**

Put the oats in a bowl, add the milk and leave to soak
overnight in the refrigerator. Keep the fruit, yogurt
and fromage frais in the refrigerator overnight.

In the morning, chop the bananas and place in a
blender with all the remaining ingredients. Blend
until smooth, then pass through a fine sieve and
serve in iced glasses, with more ice and straws.

Rating: ♥ ♥ 🍎🍎

Champneys fresh yogurt muesli

Serves 4

2 tablespoons **rolled oats**
1 tablespoon **oatbran**
1 tablespoon **wheatgerm**
about 100 ml/3^1/$_2$ fl oz **skimmed milk**
2 tablespoons **chopped mixed nuts**
3 **dried apricots**
1 **red apple**, coarsely grated
1 **green apple**, coarsely grated
1 **banana**, diced
grated zest of 1 **orange**
200 ml/7 fl oz **low-fat Greek yogurt**
1 tablespoon **maple syrup**
200 g/7 oz **fresh berries**
sprigs of **mint**, to decorate

Put the oats, oatbran and wheatgerm in a large bowl, add enough milk to cover and leave to soak overnight in the refrigerator.

In the morning, add all the remaining ingredients and mix together, stirring in the delicate berry fruits last. Serve in bowls or elegant glasses and decorate with sprigs of mint.

Rating: ♥ ♥ 🍎🍎🍎

Bulgar wheat, apple, pear and cinnamon muesli

Serves 4

50 g/2 oz **bulgar wheat**
50 g/2 oz **sugar**
1 teaspoon **ground cinnamon**
1/2 teaspoon **ground ginger**
grated zest and juice of 1 **orange**
200 ml/7 fl oz **soya milk**
40 g/11/2 oz whole **almonds**, plus extra to serve
1 **red apple**, diced
1 **green apple**, diced
1 ripe **pear**, diced
2 tablespoons **clear honey**
100 g/31/2 oz **blackcurrants**
icing sugar and sprigs of **mint**, to decorate

Put the bulgar wheat, sugar, cinnamon, ginger, orange zest and juice and soya milk in a small saucepan. Bring to the boil and simmer until the bulgar wheat has absorbed all the milk. Leave to cool and then mix with the almonds and diced apples and pear.

Put the honey and blackcurrants in a small saucepan, boil for 2 minutes, then leave to cool.

Serve the muesli in bowls and spoon the black-currants on top. Add a few more almonds, sprinkle with icing sugar and decorate with sprigs of mint.

Rating: ♥ ◉ 🍎🍎

SOUPS

Mushroom, butter bean and tarragon soup
Serves 4
2 large **onions**, sliced
2 garlic **cloves**, crushed
25 g/1 oz **dried ceps** (porcini mushrooms)
120 g/4 oz **flat field mushrooms**
500 ml/16 fl oz **semi-skimmed milk**
1 **bay leaf**
400 g/14 oz cooked **butter beans**
1 small bunch **tarragon**, leaves only
2 tablespoons **fromage frais**
salt and **pepper**

In a thick-bottomed, non-stick saucepan, dry-cook the onions and garlic until golden brown. Add the dried and fresh mushrooms, the milk, bay leaf and butter beans and simmer for 20 minutes.

Add three-quarters of the tarragon, then liquidize the soup until smooth and pass through a sieve. Whisk in half the fromage frais, season to taste with salt and pepper and reheat gently.

Chop the remaining tarragon very finely, then mix with the remaining fromage frais. Pour the hot soup into warmed bowls and swirl in the tarragon fromage frais.

Rating: ♥ ♥ 🍎🍎🍎

Lentil, lime and coriander soup

with mint and chilli yogurt

Serves 4

25 g/1 oz **puy lentils**
140 g/5 oz **red split lentils**
4 sticks **celery**, roughly chopped
1 large **onion**, roughly chopped
1 **carrot**, roughly chopped
1 **red pepper**, deseeded and roughly chopped
2 **garlic cloves**
500 ml/16 fl oz **vegetable stock**
3 **bay leaves**
finely grated zest and juice of 1 **lime**
1/2 teaspoon **lime pickle** (just the liquid)
2 tablespoons **tomato purée**
1 small bunch **coriander**
salt and **pepper**
2 tablespoons **low-fat Greek yogurt**
1 teaspoon chopped **mint** or 1/4 teaspoon **mint
  sauce concentrate** or 1 teaspoon **mint jelly**
1/2 teaspoon **sweet chilli sauce**

Put the puy lentils in a saucepan, cover with cold water
and bring to the boil. Cook for 20 minutes until tender, then drain and set aside. Cook the red lentils in a
separate saucepan for 15 minutes, then drain.

In a large saucepan, dry-cook the celery, onion, carrot, red pepper and garlic over a low heat, stirring constantly for 5 minutes. Then add the stock, bay leaves,
lime zest, lime pickle, tomato purée and the cooked
red lentils. Bring to a simmer and cook over a low heat
for 30 minutes until all the vegetables are tender.

Remove the bay leaves. Add the coriander leaves and liquidize until smooth, then pass through a sieve into another pan.

Add the cooked puy lentils and season to taste with the lime juice, salt and pepper. Mix the yogurt with the mint and sweet chilli sauce. To serve, gently reheat the soup and serve in warmed bowls, with the mint and chilli yogurt on top.

Rating: ♥ ♥ 🍎🍎🍎

Carrot, peanut, orange and sesame soup

Serves 4

500 g/1lb 2 oz **carrots**, roughly chopped
2 small **onions**, roughly chopped
1 **leek**, roughly chopped
4 sticks **celery**, roughly chopped
2 **garlic cloves**
750 ml/1¼ pints **chicken** or **vegetable stock**
finely grated zest and juice of 1 **orange**
100 g/3½ oz cooked **butter beans**
100 ml/3½ fl oz **semi-skimmed milk**
1 **bay leaf**
1 teaspoon chopped **tarragon**
2 tablespoons **peanut butter**
1 teaspoon **tahini**
½ teaspoon **sesame seeds**, toasted

Heat the oven to 200°C/400°F/gas 6. Roast the carrots, onions, leek, celery and garlic in a non-stick roasting tin for 20 minutes until golden brown.

Transfer the roasted vegetables to a saucepan and

add the stock, orange juice, butter beans, milk, bay leaf and tarragon. Bring to the boil and simmer for 10-15 minutes. Add the orange zest, peanut butter and tahini.

Liquidize until smooth and then pass through a sieve. Serve in bowls, sprinkled with the sesame seeds.

Rating: ♥ ♥ 🍎🍎🍎

Clear chicken soup
with chicken, prawn and ginger dim sum
Serves 4
750 ml/1¼ pints **chicken stock**
1-2 teaspoons **soy sauce**
1 teaspoon **rice wine**
1 teaspoon **sesame oil**
25 g/1 oz **beansprouts**
2 **pak choi**, shredded
1 **carrot**, cut into fine strips
8 fresh **shiitake mushrooms**, sliced

Dim sum:
1 **garlic clove**, crushed
1 teaspoon grated **fresh ginger**
1 teaspoon each of **plum sauce**, **soy sauce** and **thai fish sauce**
pinch of **chilli powder**
pinch of **five-spice powder**
1 bunch **spring onions**, chopped
¹/2 **egg white**
200 g/7 oz **chicken breast**, skin removed, finely chopped

90 g/3 oz cooked **prawns**, finely chopped
90 g/3 oz **fine egg noodles**

To make the dim sum, mix the garlic, ginger, plum sauce, soy sauce, fish sauce, chilli powder, five-spice powder, half the chopped spring onions and the 1/2 egg white together in a bowl. Stir in the chopped chicken and prawns. Leave to marinate in the refrigerator for 1-2 hours.

Soak the noodles or cook them according to the packet instructions. Drain on kitchen paper. To shape the dim sum, roll the chicken and prawn mixture into small, walnut-sized balls; you will need 12 in total. Lay out 6 or 7 noodles side by side and cut into 20cm/8 inch lengths. Roll each chicken and prawn ball over the top of the noodles so that the ball is wrapped in noodles. Keep on a tray in the refrigerator until ready to use.

For the soup, put the chicken stock in a saucepan with 1 teaspoon of the soy sauce and the rice wine and bring to the boil. Heat the sesame oil in a wok or non-stick frying pan and stir-fry the vegetables, adding a splash or two of water to prevent sticking. Add to the soup and boil for 2 minutes. Taste the soup and add a little more soy sauce if you like.

To serve, steam the dim sum in a bamboo steamer over a saucepan of boiling water for 3-4 minutes. Ladle the soup and vegetables into soup bowls. Add 3 steamed dim sum to each plate, sprinkle with the remaining spring onions and serve hot.

Rating: ♥ ♥ 🍎🍎

STARTERS

Grilled lobster tails

with ratatouille, spinach and basil

Serves 4

4 x 100 g/3^{1}/2 oz raw **lobster tails**, shells removed

sea salt and freshly ground **black pepper**

cooking oil in a spray can

200 g/7 oz **baby spinach**

20 **basil leaves**

^{1}/2 **lemon**

Roasted red pepper dressing (see page 205)

Ratatouille:

2 **garlic cloves**, finely chopped

100 ml/ 3^{1}/2 fl oz **dry white wine**

1 teaspoon chopped **basil**

1 small **aubergine**, cut into 2 cm/ ^{3}/4 inch dice

2 tablespoons **extra virgin olive oil**

2 **red onions**, cut into 1 cm/ ^{1}/2 inch dice

1 **red**, 1 **green** and 1 **yellow pepper**, cut into 2 cm/ ^{1}/2 inch dice

2 **courgettes**, cut into 2cm/ ^{3}/4 inch dice

6 tablespoons **tomato passata**

1 tablespoon **balsamic vinegar**

1 tablespoon **honey**

6 **tomatoes**, skinned, deseeded and cut into 1 cm/ ^{1}/2 inch dice

1 tablespoon chopped **parsley**

Heat the oven to 180°C/350°F/gas 4. For the ratatouille, liquidize 1 garlic clove with the white wine, basil, 3 tablespoons water, salt and pepper. Mix with the diced aubergine, place in a roasting tin and cook for 20-25 minutes until soft.

Heat a thick-bottomed saucepan, add 1 tablespoon olive oil, then add the onions and cook over low heat until they caramelize; remove from the pan. Add the remaining olive oil to the pan and heat until smoking. Fry the peppers for 2 minutes until well browned, then remove and add to the onions. Fry the courgettes for 2-3 minutes until well browned, then add to the onions and peppers. Return the onions, peppers and courgettes to the pan, add the cooked aubergine, the remaining garlic clove, passata, balsamic vinegar and honey and cook slowly for 20-30 minutes until it thickens. Add the tomato and parsley to the ratatouille and cook for 4 minutes, then season to taste.

Season the lobster tails with sea salt and black pepper. Heat a non-stick griddle pan over high heat, spray with a little oil and griddle the lobster for 2-3 minutes on each side.

In a saucepan over high heat, wilt the spinach with the basil for $1^1/_2$ minutes, then remove with a slotted spoon and place in the centre of 4 serving plates; season with salt and pepper. Spoon the ratatouille over the spinach and serve a lobster tail on top of the ratatouille. Squeeze a little lemon juice over the lobster and serve with a little roasted pepper dressing.

Rating: ♥ ♡ 🍎🍎🍎

Variation: Use king prawns instead of lobster tails.

Marinated sardine fillets

with leeks and red pepper mayonnaise

Serves 4

1 small bunch **basil**

3 tablespoons **extra virgin olive oil**

2 tablespoons finely chopped **parsley**

2 tablespoons finely chopped **coriander**

1 1/2 tablespoons finely chopped **oregano**

1 teaspoon **caster sugar**

2 tablespoons **white wine**

juice of 1 **lime** (or 2 if small)

salt and **pepper**

8 **sardines**, filleted

2 small **leeks**, finely sliced

Red pepper mayonnaise:

1 large **potato**, cooked

1 **red pepper**, roasted, skinned and deseeded

1/2 small **red chilli**, deseeded and ground in a mortar
   and pestle

2 tablespoons **extra virgin olive oil**

1 tablespoon **fromage frais**

Blanch the basil in boiling water for 10 seconds and
then refresh in ice-cold water. Liquidize the basil
thoroughly with 2 tablespoons of the olive oil, then
leave to drip through a coffee filter into a clean bowl;
do not press or the oil will become cloudy.

Mix the parsley, coriander and oregano with the
sugar, wine, lime juice, 1 tablespoon olive oil, salt
and pepper in a shallow dish. Take out one-third of
the mixture and place in a bowl. Grill the sardine

fillets, skin side up, on a non-stick roasting tin for 3 minutes, then put them in the shallow dish with the herb mixture. Steam the leeks for 3 minutes, then put them in the bowl with the herb mixture. Leave the sardines and leeks to marinate in the herb mixture; this could be made a day ahead.

In a food processor, liquidize the potato, red pepper, chilli, olive oil and fromage frais until thick and smooth, like mayonnaise. Season to taste with salt, then pass through a fine sieve.

Serve the sardine fillets and leeks on top of the mayonnaise and squeeze a little lime juice on top. Drizzle the basil oil around the plate.

Rating: ♥ ♡ 🍎🍎

Roasted monkfish tail

on a green bean and olive salad
Serves 4
3 tablespoons **dry white wine**
1 **garlic clove**, finely chopped
grated zest and juice of 1 **lemon**
1 teaspoon **caster sugar**
1 teaspoon crushed **coriander seeds**
sea salt and freshly ground **black pepper**
1 **monkfish tail** (about 450 g/1 lb), boned and cut
  into eight strips
1 **red onion**, cut into 8 wedges

Green bean salad:
juice of 1/2 **lemon**
1 tablespoon **white wine vinegar**

1 teaspoon **caster sugar**

1 teaspoon **dijon mustard**

2 tablespoons **extra virgin olive oil**

1 tablespoon chopped **chervil**

1 tablespoon chopped **basil**

1 tablespoon chopped **parsley**

1 tablespoon chopped **fennel herb**

1/4 **red onion**, finely chopped

200 g/7 oz **green beans**

3 **tomatoes**, skinned, deseeded and cut into batons

8 **black olives**, pitted and halved

First make the salad; whisk together the lemon juice, vinegar, sugar, mustard, olive oil and a little salt and pepper, then add the herbs and onion. Blanch the beans in salted boiling water for 4 minutes, then drain and refresh in cold water. Drain well, pat dry on kitchen paper and add the herb dressing, together with the tomatoes. Leave to marinate for 2 hours.

Mix the wine, garlic, lemon zest and juice, sugar, coriander, salt and pepper in a shallow dish, add the monkfish and leave to marinate for 1 hour.

Heat the oven to 230°C/450°F/gas 8. Put the onion wedges in a small roasting tin lined with baking parchment and roast for 15 minutes until tender and browned.

To cook the monkfish, heat a non-stick frying pan over high heat, add the monkfish and turn to seal all over. Continue cooking for 5-6 minutes until golden brown, but still moist in the centre.

While the fish is cooking, strain the bean salad over a jug. Pile the salad in the centre of 4 serving plates. Put the roasted red onion wedges on top and then the monkfish. Add the strained bean salad dressing to the frying pan together with the olives. Warm gently and pour over the fish. Serve warm.

Rating: ♥ ♡ 🍎🍎

Variation: Use hake instead on monkfish.

Baked mushrooms
with broccoli and apricot pesto
Serves 4
8 **fresh red chillies**, deseeded and cut into 2 cm/ ³/4 inch pieces
4 large **flat mushrooms**
juice of ¹/2 **orange**
2 tablespoons **walnut oil**
¹/2 teaspoon **tarragon mustard**
1 tablespoon **fromage frais**
2 **tomatoes**, skinned, deseeded and diced
50 g/2 oz **corn salad**
15 g/¹/2 oz mixed **fresh herbs** (chervil, coriander, flat-leaf parsley)

Broccoli and apricot pesto:
500 g/1 lb 2oz **broccoli**
1 **garlic clove**, crushed
2 tablespoons **dry sherry**
2 tablespoons grated **parmesan cheese**
1 tablespoon **fromage frais**
freshly ground **black pepper**
6 **dried apricots**, chopped

Heat the oven to 200°C/400°F/gas 6. Place the chillies on a non-stick baking sheet and roast for 7-8 minutes; this will intensify the flavour and remove most of the heat from the chillies.

Peel the mushrooms; cut off and discard the stalks. Slice each mushroom very thinly horizontally to make 3 or 4 circular slices from each mushroom.

To make the pesto: using a sharp knife, shave the flowering tops of the broccoli, being careful not to take too much of the stalk. (You will end up with around 120 g/4 oz of broccoli tops.) Heat a small saucepan and add the garlic and broccoli tops. Cook for 30 seconds, then coat with the dry sherry. Remove from the heat and add the Parmesan, fromage frais and a good grinding of black pepper. Add the apricots and blend with a hand-held blender until smooth. Reduce the oven temperature to 190°C/ 375°F/gas 5. Re-form the mushrooms by layering the slices with a little of the pesto, reserving some of the pesto to serve. If you like, use a large pastry cutter to trim the mushrooms to a uniform size. Place on a non-stick roasting tin and bake for 20 minutes.

Blend a quarter of the roasted chillies with the orange juice, walnut oil, tarragon mustard and romage frais. Pass through a fine sieve. Dice the remaining chillies and mix with the diced tomatoes, corn salad and herbs.

Serve the mushrooms hot or cold. Arrange the salad in the centre of 4 plates and dress with a little of the chilli dressing. Place the mushrooms on the salad and top with a little pesto.

Rating: ♥ ♥ 🍎🍎🍎

Carpaccio of tuna

with ginger and sesame salad

Serves 4

4 x 70 g/2$\frac{1}{2}$ oz perfectly fresh **yellowfin tuna steaks**, each 2 cm/$\frac{3}{4}$ inch thick

1 teaspoon **groundnut oil** for brushing cling film

$\frac{1}{2}$ teaspoon **caster sugar**

$\frac{1}{2}$ teaspoon very finely chopped **fresh ginger**

$\frac{1}{2}$ teaspoon very finely chopped **red** or **green chilli**

1 teaspoon **sesame oil**

1 teaspoon **sesame seeds**, toasted

sea salt

1 **lime**, halved

100 g/3$\frac{1}{2}$ oz mixed **curly endive** (frisée) and **sprouting beans** and **lentils** (alfalfa, mung beans, chickpeas)

To prepare the tuna, place each steak between two pieces of lightly oiled cling film and beat gently with a rolling pin until it is 2 mm/$\frac{1}{8}$ inch thick – be very careful and keep turning the tuna so that you finish with a neat round shape without holes. Leave in the cling film and keep in the refrigerator until ready to serve.

Make the dressing in advance as it will improve in flavour. Whisk together the sugar, ginger, chilli and sesame oil, then stir in the toasted sesame seeds and a little sea salt.

To serve, peel one side of the cling film off the tuna and lay face down on a cold serving plate, then carefully remove the other piece of cling film. Squeeze the lime juice over the tuna. Dress the salad leaves and sprouts with a little of the dressing and pile in the centre of the tuna. Sprinkle the remaining dressing over the tuna.

Rating: ♥ 🅥 🍎🍎

Variation: If you do not like uncooked tuna, you can follow the recipe but grill the fish under a high heat.

Aubergine cannelloni
with courgette and smoked salmon and provençal sauce
Serves 4
2 large **aubergines**
2 **courgettes**
1 **garlic clove**, finely chopped
grated zest of 1/4 **lemon** and juice of 11/2 **lemons**
3 tablespoons **dry white wine**
3 tablespoons **olive oil**
4 teaspoons **caster sugar**
salt and freshly ground **black pepper**
36 **basil leaves**
140 g/5 oz sliced **smoked salmon**
15 g/1/2 oz **chives**, chopped
140 g/5 oz **cottage cheese**
3 tablespoons **fromage frais**
1 tablespoon **pine nuts**, toasted
100 g/31/2 oz baby **spinach**

Provençal sauce:
1 **red onion**, finely chopped
1/2 **garlic clove**, finely chopped

1 tablespoon **olive oil**
3 tablespoons **balsamic vinegar**
1 teaspoon **caster sugar**
6 tablespoons **tomato passata**
1 **red**, 1 **green** and 1 **yellow pepper**, roasted,
   skinned, deseeded and diced
4 **tomatoes**, skinned, deseeded and diced
dash of **sweet chilli sauce**

Heat the oven to 190°C/375°F/gas 5. Cut the
aubergines lengthways into very thin slices (about
1mm thick), discarding the other pieces (you should
have 12 slices). Lay the slices on a baking sheet lined
with baking parchment. Do the same with the
courgettes. Mix the garlic with the juice of 1 lemon,
the wine, 2 tablespoons olive oil, 3 teaspoons sugar,
salt and pepper, blend with a hand-held blender and
then brush on to the aubergine and courgette slices.
Bake for 10-15 minutes until tender. While still warm
lay 3 leaves of basil on each slice of aubergine and
then lay a slice of courgette on top and leave to cool
slightly. This will release the oils from the basil into
the aubergine.

Cut the smoked salmon into strips of a similar size
to the courgette slices and lay a piece of salmon on
top of each. Mix the chives with the cottage cheese,
fromage frais and pine nuts and season to taste with a
small amount of salt and lots of black pepper. Spread
on to the smoked salmon and then roll up into 12
rolls.

To make the sauce, soften the onion and garlic in
the olive oil over a low heat. Add the balsamic vinegar

and sugar and simmer until reduced by half. Add the passata, peppers and tomatoes and cook for 2 minutes. Season to taste with salt, pepper and a dash of sweet chilli sauce.

Whisk the remaining lemon juice with the zest, the remaining 1 tablespoon olive oil and 1 teaspoon sugar, salt and pepper to taste. Toss the spinach in the lemon vinaigrette and then sauté for 30 seconds until just beginning to wilt. Serve the aubergine cannelloni with the warm spinach and Provençal sauce. This could also be served cold.

Rating: ♥ ♡ 🍎🍎🍎

MAIN COURSES

Beans on toast
with melted smoked goats' cheese
Serves 4
50 g/2 oz cooked **borlotti beans**
50 g/2 oz cooked **flageolet beans**
50 g/2 oz cooked **haricot beans**
50 g/2 oz cooked **blackeye beans**
50 g/2 oz cooked **kidney beans**
4 thick slices **wholemeal bread**, lightly toasted
   on both sides
90 g/3 oz **smoked** (or unsmoked) **goats' cheese**,
   cut into 4 slices

Tomato sauce:
500 g/1 lb 2 oz ripe **tomatoes**
2 small **onions**, chopped
6 **garlic cloves**, roasted then peeled
1 tablespoon **tomato purée**
3 tablespoons **dry white wine**
150 ml/5 fl oz **vegetable stock**
2 **bay leaves**
pinch of **ground cumin**
pinch of **paprika**
pinch of **chilli powder**
2 tablespoons **sugar**
1 tablespoon **olive oil**
1 **red pepper**, roasted, skinned, deseeded and diced
salt and **pepper**

To cook the pulses, if using dried, soak in cold water

for at least 8 hours, then drain and cover with fresh cold water. Bring to the boil and boil for 2-3 hours; do not add salt as this will make the skins tough and inhibit the beans from cooking all the way through. If using tinned beans, just rinse and set aside.

For the tomato sauce, heat the oven to 220°C/425°F/gas 7. Cut 400 g/14 oz of the tomatoes in half. Squeeze out the seeds, then roast the tomatoes in the oven for 15 minutes. Blanch, peel, deseed an dice the remaining tomatoes and set aside.

In a thick-bottomed saucepan, dry-cook three-quarters of the chopped onion with the roasted garlic, tomato purée and roasted tomatoes. Add the wine, stock, bay leaves, cumin, paprika, chilli powder and sugar and cook very slowly over a low heat until the mixture has reduced by two-thirds.

Meanwhile, in a separate saucepan, cook the remaining onion in the olive oil over a low heat until the onion caramelizes.

Add the cooked beans to the caramelized onion. Pass the tomato mixture through a sieve and add to the beans. Simmer on a low heat for 20-30 minutes until the beans have absorbed the tomato sauce.

Add the diced tomato and pepper to the beans. Season to taste with a little salt and pepper and spoon on to the toasted bread, making sure that the toast is totally covered with the beans so that the edges do not burn. Lay the goats' cheese on top and place under a very hot grill until golden brown.

Rating: ♥ ♥ 🍅🍅🍅

Grilled aubergine parcels

with goats' cheese, tomatoes, olives and basil

Serves 4

2 large **aubergines**, topped and tailed

1 large **onion**, chopped

4 **garlic cloves**: 2 finely chopped, 2 sliced

200 g/7 oz canned chopped **tomatoes**

100 g/3½ oz soft **goats' cheese** kept in the freezer
    for 15-20 minutes to make it easier to cut, then
    sliced into 8

1 bunch **basil**

16 **black olives**, pitted

2 tablespoons **olive oil**

juice of 1 **lemon**

sea salt and freshly ground **black pepper**

140 g/5 oz **cherry tomatoes**, red and yellow

4 **shallots**, sliced

25 g/1 oz **pine nuts**, toasted

Slice the aubergines lengthways as thinly as possible
with a very sharp knife or a mandolin slicer. You will
need 4 slices per person. Cook the aubergines in a large
saucepan of salted boiling water for 2 minutes, then
refresh under cold water and drain on kitchen paper.

Put the onion and chopped garlic into a saucepan
and then strain the juice of the tomatoes on top.
Cook over a high heat until reduced by two-thirds.
Then add the chopped tomatoes, reduce the heat
slightly and continue cooking for about 5 minutes or
until the mixture is quite dry. Leave to cool.

Lay a slice of aubergine on a chopping board and
then lay another slice across the centre to make a

cross shape. Put a piece of goats' cheese in the centre of the aubergine cross, then add a little of the tomato and onion mixture, a couple of fresh basil leaves and then 2 olives and a little more tomato and onion mixture and basil. Fold the aubergine ends in to the centre to form a parcel. Repeat with the remaining aubergine slices until you have 8 parcels.

Heat the oven to 220°C/425°F/gas 7. Heat a griddle pan over a high heat. Mix 1 tablespoon of olive oil with the lemon juice, salt and pepper; brush this mixture over the aubergine parcels. Cook the parcels on the griddle pan for 1 minute on each side, then place in the oven for 6-8 minutes. Put the whole cherry tomatoes, the sliced shallots and sliced garlic in a small roasting tin with 1 tablespoon olive oil and roast for 5 minutes.

Serve 2 aubergine parcels per person, with a spoonful of the roasted cherry tomato and shallot mixture, a few pine nuts and a few sprigs of basil.

Rating: ♥ ♥ 🍎🍎🍎

Refried bean and avocado cakes
with avocado and corn salsa
Serves 4
200 g/7 oz **red kidney beans**, soaked overnight and
   cooked until tender
1 red **chilli**, deseeded and chopped
4 **garlic cloves**, roasted
pinch of crushed, roasted **coriander seeds**
pinch of **ground cumin**
juice of 1 **lime**, plus 1 **lime**, quartered, to serve

50 g/2 oz **low-fat cheddar cheese**, grated
6 **shallots**, finely chopped
1/2 **avocado**, finely diced
sea salt and **pepper**
2 tablespoons **low-fat crème fraîche**

Avocado and corn salsa:
50 g/2 oz frozen **sweetcorn kernels**, thawed
1 small **onion**, chopped
1 **tomato**, skinned, deseeded and diced
2 teaspoons **sweet chilli sauce**
1 bunch **coriander**, leaves roughly torn
1/2 **avocado**, diced
juice of 2 **limes**

Drain the beans and pat dry with kitchen paper.
Mash the beans to a paste with a potato masher. With
a pestle and mortar, crush the fresh chilli with the
roasted garlic, coriander seeds and cumin. Add the
juice of 1 lime and mix with the beans. Add the
grated cheese, shallots and diced avocado and mix
carefully so that you do not crush the avocado.
Season to taste with salt and pepper. Divide the
mixture into 8 balls, then, using your hands, form
into cakes approximately 1cm/1/2inch thick. Place on
a baking sheet lined with baking parchment and
refrigerate until ready to cook.

To make the salsa, toast the sweetcorn in a non-
stick pan over a high heat. It is important that you
keep stirring so that the sweetcorn colours evenly.
When the sweetcorn is toasted, mix with the onion,
tomato, sweet chilli sauce and coriander. Finally, stir

in the avocado and lime juice and season to taste with a little salt.

To serve, heat the oven to 200°C/400°F/gas 6. Bake the bean cakes for approximately 15 minutes, turning after 7 minutes, until they are evenly coloured.

Serve the hot bean cakes on the cold salsa, add a little low-fat crème fraîche and a lime quarter and serve at once.

Rating: ♥ ♥ 🍎🍎🍎

SALADS

Champneys salad niçoise
Serves 4
200 g/7 oz **swordfish**, very thinly sliced
100 g/3^1/$_2$ oz **sugar snap peas**
100 g/3^1/$_2$ oz **mangetout**
12 **black olives**, halved
1 **red onion**, chopped
2 **beef tomatoes**, skinned, deseeded and diced
4 **salad potatoes**, cooked and diced
100 g/3^1/$_2$ oz **baby spinach leaves**
1 teaspoon chopped **flat-leaf parsley**

Dressing:
1 tablespoon **anchovy essence**
^{1}/$_2$ teaspoon **dijon mustard**
^{1}/$_2$ teaspoon **sugar**
1 teaspoon **red wine vinegar**
1 teaspoon **chopped capers**
1 tablespoon **extra virgin olive oil**

To make the dressing, whisk the anchovy essence with the mustard, sugar, vinegar and capers. Finally whisk in the olive oil.

Heat the grill. Cook the swordfish on a non-stick baking sheet under the hot grill for about 5 minutes on each side. Leave to cool in the dressing.

Cook the sugar snap peas in salted boiling water for 1 minute, then drain and refresh in ice-cold water. Blanch the mangetout in salted boiling water, then drain, refresh and cut diagonally. Gently toss the peas and mangetout with all the remaining salad ingredients and serve between layers of swordfish.

Rating: ♥ ⊘ 🍎🍎🍎
Variation: Use tuna instead of swordfish.

Fennel, asparagus and walnut salad
with orange mayonnaise
Serves 4
2 **fennel bulbs**, thinly sliced
1 bunch **asparagus**, trimmed and cut into
   3 cm/1 inch pieces
1 **curly endive** (frisée)
6 **walnuts**, roasted and chopped into
   5 mm/ $^1/4$ inch pieces
4 tablespoons **chopped mixed herbs** (parsley,
   chervil, coriander)
juice of 1 **orange**
peppercorns (preferably Szechwan), in a pepper
mill

Orange mayonnaise:
2 **potatoes**, peeled, diced and cooked until tender
finely grated zest and juice of 2 **oranges**
2 tablespoons **fromage frais**
1 tablespoon **low-fat yogurt**
2 tablespoons **walnut oil**
salt and **pepper**

To make the orange mayonnaise, put the potatoes, orange zest and juice, fromage frais, yogurt and walnut oil in a food processor. Blend until smooth, season to taste with salt and pepper, then pass through a fine sieve.

Steam the fennel for 2 minutes, then set aside. Steam the asparagus for 2 minutes, refresh in ice-cold water, then drain. Pick the heart of the curly endive into small pieces and mix with the walnuts and the herbs. Toss in the orange juice. Pile the leafy salad in the centre of the serving dish and pile the steamed asparagus and fennel on top. Spoon over the orange mayonnaise and grind some pepper coarsely over the top.

Rating: ♥ ♥ 🍎🍎🍎

Salad of tomatoes and eggs
with parmesan crisps
Serves 4
50 g/2 oz **parmesan cheese**, freshly grated
4 fresh **eggs**
1 tablespoon **white wine vinegar**
10 **yellow cherry tomatoes**
10 **red cherry tomatoes**
50 g/2 oz **baby spinach leaves**
50 g/2 oz **baby red chard** or **beetroot leaves**
a few **baby basil leaves**

Sun-dried tomato dressing:
6 **sun-dried tomatoes**
2 tablespoons **balsamic vinegar**
2 tablespoons **extra virgin olive oil**
1/2 teaspoon **sugar**
1 small cooked **potato**
salt and freshly ground **black pepper**

Heat the oven to 190°C/375°F/gas 5. To make the Parmesan crisps, sprinkle the Parmesan in a thin, even layer (less than 1 mm thick) in 8 rough triangle shapes on a non-stick baking sheet. (You can make a template by cutting triangles out of an old plastic lid, using a sharp knife.) Bake for 4-6 minutes until golden brown. When cooked, loosen them carefully with a palette knife and leave to cool on the baking sheet. These crisps can be made in advance and kept in an airtight container until ready to use.

To cook the eggs, carefully break them into gently simmering water to which you have added the vinegar. The eggs will take about 3-4 minutes to cook and should be softly poached. Plunge into iced water to prevent them from over-cooking.

To make the dressing, liquidize the sun-dried tomatoes with the balsamic vinegar, olive oil, sugar, potato and 4 tablespoons cold water until smooth, then pass through a fine sieve. Season to taste; this dressing will probably not need any salt because of the sun-dried tomatoes, but use lots of black pepper.

To assemble the salad, cut the tomatoes in half and then mix with the salad leaves and drizzle with the dressing. Place in the centre of the serving plates. Drain the poached eggs on kitchen paper and place on the salad. Serve the Parmesan crisps on top.

Rating: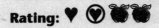

Bean salad

with roasted cherry tomatoes and avocado salsa

Serves 4

20 **cherry tomatoes**
50 g/2 oz **runner beans**, cut into strips
50 g/2 oz **french beans**, cut into 3 cm/1 inch lengths
50 g/2 oz cooked **red kidney beans**
50 g/2 oz cooked **broad beans**, skinned
50 g/2 oz cooked **haricot beans**

Avocado salsa:

1 teaspoon **coriander seeds**, roasted and crushed
1 **garlic clove**, crushed
1 bunch **coriander**, chopped
1 teaspoon **sugar**
finely grated zest and juice of 4 **limes**
1/2 **green leek**, finely chopped
4 **shallots**, finely chopped
1 small **green chilli pepper**, finely chopped
1 **green pepper**, cut into 5 mm/1/4 inch dice
salt
1 **avocado**, cut into 5 mm/1/4 inch dice

To make the avocado salsa, mix the coriander seeds
with the garlic, most of the chopped coriander
(reserving a little for garnish), sugar, lime zest and
juice, leek, shallots, chilli and green pepper. Season to
taste with a little salt and refrigerate for at least 4
hours.

Heat the oven to 200°C/400°F/gas 6. Put the cherry
tomatoes in a small roasting tin and roast for about
10 minutes until they just begin to char and collapse.

Leave to cool.

Meanwhile, blanch the runner beans and French beans in boiling water for 1 minute. Drain and refresh in ice-cold water.

Mix all the beans together, mix with the salsa and add the diced avocado. Leave for at least 2 hours to let the flavours develop.

Serve the bean salad on top of the tomatoes and garnish with fresh coriander.

Rating: ♥ ♥ 🍎🍎🍎

DRESSINGS

All dressing recipes serve 10-12 and can be kept in the refrigerator for 3-4 days. Ideally, ingredients should be liquidized with a hand-held blender.

Fat-free fresh herb and roasted garlic dressing

3 cloves **garlic**, sliced
1 small **potato** (about 25 g/1 oz), cooked
1 teaspoon crushed **coriander seeds**
1 tablespoon chopped **parsley**
1 tablespoon chopped **coriander**
1 tablespoon chopped **dill**
1 tablespoon chopped **chervil**
1 tablespoon chopped **chives**
3 tablespoons **dry white wine**
1 teaspoon **white wine vinegar**
1/2 teaspoon **tarragon vinegar**
3 tablespoons **water**
salt and freshly ground **black pepper**

Spread the garlic on a baking sheet and roast under a low grill for 5-6 minutes until lightly browned.

Liquidize all the ingredients, then push through a fine sieve. Season to taste.

Rating: 🍎

Sun-dried tomato, olive and rosemary dressing

50 g/2 oz **sun-dried tomatoes**, soaked in boiling water for 20 minutes, then drained
2 sprigs of **rosemary**, leaves stripped from the stalks
1 small **new potato**, cooked
2 tablespoon pitted and chopped **green olives**
1 **garlic clove**, peeled
3 tablespoons **extra virgin olive oil**
2 tablespoons **balsamic vinegar**
1/2 teaspoon **dijon mustard**
6 tablespoons **water**
salt and freshly ground **black pepper**

Liquidize all the ingredients until smooth, then pass through a fine sieve and season to taste with salt and pepper.

Rating:

Fat-free roasted red pepper, chilli and rosemary dressing

1 large **red pepper**
1 **red chilli pepper**, cut in half, deseeded and cored
1 small **potato** (about 25 g/1 oz)
1/2 clove **garlic**
1 teaspoon **clear honey**
1 tablespoon chopped **rosemary**
1 teaspoon **English mustard**
juice of 1/2 **lemon**

1 teaspoon **white wine vinegar**
salt and freshly ground **black pepper**

Heat the oven to 230ºC/450ºF/gas 8. Put the pepper, chilli and potato on a baking sheet and roast in the hot oven until the pepper skin is blackened and the potato is cooked. Halve the pepper over a plate to collect the juice. Pull off the stalk and scrape out the seeds.

Liquidize the pepper with all the remaining ingredients, then pass through a fine sieve. Season to taste with salt and pepper.

Rating:

DESSERT

Iced apricot mousse
with pistachios and warm plum compote
Serves 4
200 g/7 oz **dried apricots**
grated zest and juice of 1 **orange**
2 tablespoons **fromage frais**
2 tablespoons **thick low-fat yogurt**
2 tablespoons **low-fat crème fraîche**
1 **vanilla pod**
2 **egg whites**
50 g/2 oz **pistachio nuts**, blanched, peeled and
  finely chopped

Plum compote:
12 **plums**, cut in half, stones removed
2 slices of **stem ginger** preserved in syrup, diced,
plus 2 tablespoons of the **ginger syrup**
1/2 teaspoon **ground ginger**
2 tablespoons **brandy**
1/2 teaspoon **arrowroot**

Simmer the apricots in boiling water for 20 minutes,
then liquidize with a hand-held blender. Remove 4
tablespoons of the mixture and put into a saucepan
with half the orange juice and all the zest and cook
over a low heat for 4 minutes until thick, then pass
through a fine sieve and leave to cool.

  Mix the remaining apricot mixture with the
fromage frais, yogurt and crème fraîche. Split the
vanilla pod and scrape the seeds into the apricot

mixture. Whisk the egg whites until soft peaks form, then fold into the apricot mixture with a metal spoon, pour into 4 individual gateau rings or ramekins on a baking sheet and put into the freezer for 4 hours.

To make the plum compote, boil the plums, ginger, ginger syrup, brandy, the remaining orange juice and 4 tablespoons water over a low heat for 10 minutes until the plums are soft but still keeping their shape. Mix the arrowroot with a little water and stir into the boiling plum mixture to thicken slightly.

Slide a warm knife around the gateau rings to remove the mousses. Roll the mousses in chopped pistachios, then place on 4 serving plates. Spoon the apricot and orange sauce over the mousse and serve the warm plums around the outside.

Rating:

CHAPTER 9

THE USEFUL PAGES

Here you'll find charts to help you keep track of your achievements, a method all the *Fit Club* experts recommend. By comparing how you are progressing, you will see for yourself just how much you are improving in your exercises, and how much weight you are losing. We've also pulled together contacts you might find useful for both equipment and weightloss information.

Your achievement charts

Weight
Try to weigh yourself no more than once a week; your weight can fluctuate from day to day and it can be demotivating if water retention for example gives you a distorted reading. Weigh yourself at the same time of day: first thing in the morning before breakfast, and after going to the lavatory, is best. Either wear the same clothes each time or preferably wear nothing at all. *Celebrity Fit Club* took six months, but don't stop there on the chart!

	Weight in kilos/lbs	Weekly weightloss
Week 1		
Week 2		
Week 3		
Week 4		
Week 5		
Week 6		
Week 7		
Week 8		
Week 9		
Week 10		
Week 11		
Week 12		

	Weight in kilos/lbs	Weekly weightloss
Week 13		
Week 14		
Week 15		
Week 16		
Week 17		
Week 18		
Week 19		
Week 20		
Week 21		
Week 22		
Week 23		
Week 24		

Body measurements

Weightloss and exercise will change your shape all over. Your changing waist measurement is important because it is the most significant to your health (see pages 61-62, about pear and apple shapes), but you might want to choose an area to measure regularly.

	Waist	Hips	Chest
Week 1			
Week 2			
Week 3			
Week 4			
Week 5			
Week 6			
Week 7			
Week 8			
Week 9			
Week 10			
Week 11			
Week 12			

	Waist	Hips	Chest
Week 13			
Week 14			
Week 15			
Week 16			
Week 17			
Week 18			
Week 19			
Week 20			
Week 21			
Week 22			
Week 23			
Week 24			

Fitness achievements

Once you've chosen a form of exercise that you enjoy
and that fits in with your lifestyle, set yourself some
realistic targets to spur you on.

	Walking/ running: distance	Strengthening: repetitions	Level of exertion 1=easy 10=hard
Week 1			
Week 2			
Week 3			
Week 4			
Week 5			
Week 6			
Week 7			
Week 8			
Week 9			
Week 10			
Week 11			

	Walking/ running: distance	Strengthening: repetitions	Level of exertion 1=easy 10=hard
Week 12			
Week 13			
Week 14			
Week 15			
Week 16			
Week 17			
Week 18			
Week 19			
Week 20			
Week 21			
Week 22			
Week 23			
Week 24			

Useful information and websites

Heart-rate monitors: These are an important tool
for monitoring your pulse rate as you exercise. If your
rate is too low you will gain little from exercise; too
high and you will tire too quickly and won't burn fat.
At *Fit Club* the members used the Polar Pulse Watch
which is easy to use and water-resistant to 20m. The
watch gives high and low target zones and works
with Polar's compact (2 in 1) Waterproof Transmitter
belt. The package costs around £40.
Available from good sports shops, online from
www.premiersportsandfitness.co.uk or call Polar UK
on 01926 811711 for your nearest stockist.

Pedometers: These calculate the number of steps
you take in a day – the perfect target for an active
person or for those trying to get fit is around 10,000
per day. They are widely available (we used some
manufactured by Roche) and vary in quality, so buy
the best you can afford.

Sports bras: Large breasts can make exercise uncomfortable. The solution is a good quality sports bra
with plenty of support around the back, cup and
shoulders. Try bras from www.sportsbras.co.uk.
Another good source is Bravissimo, a company which
specializes in bras for the larger bust. Find them at
www.bravissimo.com or call 01926 459859 for a
catalogue or your nearest branch. This company also
specializes in swimwear for larger sizes.

Trainers: If you are looking for trainers in larger sizes, try www.sportsshoes.com and www.fdsports.co.uk, both of which supply shoes from size 12 to 20. Fdsports also sells XL and XXL Nike sportswear online.

Websites for support and advice on weightloss and exercise:

The Internet is a rich source of information and we have selected a group of sites which have sensible advice for anyone wanting to lose weight and become fitter. By its very nature however, the Internet has many sites which promise quick weightloss and 'fad' diets – all the elements which *Fit Club* tries to distance itself from – and you should be careful which ones you choose to browse.

About.com: www.about.com/health/ with features on weightloss, fitness and well-being.

BBC Online: www.bbc.co.uk/health/fitness/ Excellent advice on fitness for all ages.

BodySmartUK: www.bodysmartuk.com/ Personalized diet information and equipment sales online.

British Heart Foundation: www.bhf.org.uk Official site of the charity with information about healthy eating to prevent heart disease.

British Nutrition Foundation: www.nutrition.org.uk Go to nutrition facts , then to slimming diets.

Diabetes: www.diabetes.org.uk Information on this disease and early symptoms.

FeelGoodUK: www.icircle.com/ Site with a magazine style aimed at women. Gossipy but some sound advice.

Food Fitness: www.foodfitness.org.uk Site of the Food and Drink Federation; includes food and activity tips and self-assessment quiz.

Health and Fitness Magazine Online: www.hfonline.co.uk Includes an online health and training effectiveness check.

Health in Focus: www.healthinfocus.co.uk Printable health information sheets, including one on diabetes.

Health Net: www.healthnet.org.uk Site of the Coronary Prevention Group with diet and exercise information, and suggested exercises.

Mendosa.com: www.mendosa.com/gilists.htm Reliable glycaemic index lists from health writer Rick Mendosa.

Mind Body Soul: www.mindbodysoul.gov.uk Health advice for 14-16 year-olds.

NetDoctor: www.netdoctor.co.uk/health_advice/facts/loseweight.htm Online medical advice site with weightloss information.

Sports Organizations: www.sportengland.org, www.sports-council-wales.co.uk and www.sportscotland.org.uk All give information on where to get involved in a chosen sport.

Think Fast: www.thinkfast.co.uk Health Education Authority advice to help you make the healthy choice at fast food outlets, aimed at 15-34 year olds.

WeightDirectory: www.weightdirectory.com/ Good American site, with an online BMI calculator.

Weight Watchers UK: www.weightwatchers.co.uk Site has information about local meetings, and includes a BMI calculator and questionnaire to test your motivation.

Advice on eating disorders:
If you think your eating is out of control, it may help to talk to an expert.
The National Centre for Eating Disorders:
54 New Road,
Esher, Surrey KT10 9NU
01372 469493
www.eating-disorders.org.uk

The Eating Disorders Association:
First Floor, Wensum House
103 Prince of Wales Road,
Norwich NR1 1DW
Helpline: 0870 770 3221
www.edauk.com

GLOSSARY

Abdominals
Muscles in the stomach area from the ribs to the pelvis. Proper names: rectus abdominus, the obliques and the quadratus lumborum.

Aerobic Capacity
How well your body processes oxygen. This depends on your lung capacity, the size of your capillaries, the pumping action of your heart and the efficiency of oxygen transfer.

Aerobic Exercise
Low to medium-intensity long-endurance exercise when oxygen is supplied to the muscles through the blood. Involves increased heart rate and, if sustained, leads to fat burning.

Anaerobic Exercise
High intensity exercise which cannot be sustained for long. Involves the burning of carbohydrate rather than oxygen.

Basal Metabolic Rate (BMR)
Rate at which the body uses up energy when at rest. A higher proportion of lean tissue (muscle) leads to a higher BMR.

Body Fat
Fat stored within the body under the skin and around the organs.

Body Mass Index (BMI)
Calculation for working out weight levels, using height and weight in metres and kilograms.
For equation see page 56-57.

Calorie
The unit used to measure energy levels in food.
1 calorie = 4.19 kilojoules.

Carbohydrates
Nutrient made up of carbon, hydrogen and oxygen, and including lactose, glucose, starch and glycogen. Carbohydrates are found in foods based on plant products, such as vegetables, wheat and rice. Fibre is also considered to be a carbohydrate but since it cannot be digested it does not provide energy and is not considered to be a useable carbohydrate.

Cholesterol
Naturally occurring substance produced by the liver and kidneys which helps in the production of vitamin D and various hormones. Also helps absorb fatty acids. Dangerous in high amounts – caused by a diet high in saturated fats.
See page 66-68.

Dehydration
Reaction of a body that is lacking in fluids; can occur after intense exercise. Can cause headaches and dizziness.

Fats
Substance made up of fatty acids and found in foods from animals and plants. Comes in three types: saturated (usually from animal products), unsaturated (from plant foods), and essential fatty acids (usually from fish and plants).

Glucose
The simplest form of sugar, glucose occurs in some foods but is also the form of sugar that is found in

the blood. It usually results from carbohydrates being digested in the body.

Glycaemic Index

A measurement of the ability of a carbohydrate to raise glucose levels in the blood. The higher the glycaemic index, the faster the food is digested and enters the blood as glucose, thus stimulating the production of insulin. See Chapter 5.

Glycogen

The form in which carbohydrate is stored in the liver and muscles. Can be hydrolyzed into glucose.

Heart Rate

The number of beats per minute of your heart, which varies depending on the stress the body is under.

Hip to Waist Ratio

Means of calculating where fat stores are laid down in the body. See page 61-62.

Insulin

A hormone produced in the pancreas that is responsible for helping the body to burn up and store energy. When too much is produced, because of excess consumption of refined carbohydrates, it encourages the body to store it as fat.

Ketosis

Metabolic state resulting from low-carbohydrate intake, enabling the body to start burning stored fat for fuel.

Lactic Acid

Important substance in the production of energy. Builds up in the cells during high-intensity anaerobic exercise and limits sustainability, until it is recycled once enough oxygen is available.

Ligament
Band of tough fibrous tissue which connects bones
and cartilage, and supports the muscles.

Maximum Heart Rate
The maximum level at which someone should raise
their heart rate, which is calculated by 220 minus the
person's age. See page 122-123.

Metabolism
Term for the chemical changes in cells by which energy is provided for growth and body function. Resting
Metabolic Rate is the amount of energy the body
needs to keep functioning when at rest.

Muscles
Tissue in the body which can contract and expand to
allow movement. Can be toned up with exercise.

Obesity
Having excessive fat, calculated as being over 30 on
the BMI (see above).

Osteoporosis
Condition affecting the bones whereby their density
decreases and they are prone to fracture. Affects men
and women, but can be avoided with a regular exercise regime.

Pronation
Way of walking whereby the body weight is concen-
trated on the insides of the feet. See page 125.

Protein
Substances in food based on carbon, hydrogen, oxygen and nitrogen. Proteins are essential for life, building up body tissue, especially muscle, and essential
for repair, growth and energy. Extra protein is not
stored in the body so it must be eaten regularly.

Resting Pulse Rate
Number of heart beats per minute when the body is
at rest.

Supernation
Way of walking whereby the body weight is concen-
trated on the outsides of the feet. See page 125.

Tendons
Band on inelastic collagenous tissue that attaches a
muscle to the bone or other area.

Vitamins
Chemicals found in some foods essential for health,
growth and energy.